Practitioner's Guide to Developmental and Psychological Testing

CRITICAL ISSUES IN
DEVELOPMENTAL AND BEHAVIORAL PEDIATRICS

SERIES EDITOR: MARVIN I. GOTTLIEB, M.D., Ph.D.
Hackensack Medical Center
Hackensack, New Jersey
and University of Medicine and Dentistry of New Jersey—
New Jersey Medical School
Newark, New Jersey

DEVELOPMENTAL-BEHAVIORAL DISORDERS: Selected Topics
Volumes 1–3
Edited by Marvin I. Gottlieb, M.D., Ph.D., and John E. Williams, M.D.

PEDIATRIC COMPLIANCE: A Guide for the Primary Care Physician
Edward R. Christophersen, Ph.D.

PEDIATRIC ORTHOPEDICS: A Guide for the Primary Care Physician
Richard J. Mier, M.D., and Thomas D. Brower, M.D.

PRACTITIONER'S GUIDE TO DEVELOPMENTAL AND
PSYCHOLOGICAL TESTING
Glen P. Aylward, Ph.D.

A Continuation Order Plan is available for this series. A continuation order will bring delivery of each new volume immediately upon publication. Volumes are billed only upon actual shipment. For further information please contact the publisher.

Practitioner's Guide to Developmental and Psychological Testing

Glen P. Aylward, Ph.D.
Southern Illinois University School of Medicine
Springfield, Illinois

Plenum Medical Book Company
New York and London

Library of Congress Cataloging-in-Publication Data

Aylward, Glen P.
    Practitioner's guide to developmental and psychological testing /
Glen P. Aylward.
        p.   cm. -- (Critical issues in developmental and behavioral
    pediatrics)
    Includes bibliographical references and index.
    ISBN 0-306-44689-8
    1. Psychological tests for children. 2. Child development-
-Testing.   I. Title. II. Series.
    [DNLM: 1. Psychological Tests--in infancy & childhood. 2. Child
Development. 3. Achievement.   WS 105.5.E8 A9813p 1994]
RJ503.5.A94   1994
618.92'890075--dc20
DNLM/DLC
for Library of Congress   94-28015
                                                                   CIP

10 9 8 7 6 5 4 3 2

ISBN 0-306-44689-8

©1994 Plenum Publishing Corporation
233 Spring Street, New York, N.Y. 10013

Plenum Medical Book Company is an imprint of Plenum Publishing Corporation

Printed in the United States of America

To my wife and children
for their support and understanding,
and to Philip and Conner
who I wish could have seen the final product

❋ Preface

The practice of primary health care has expanded beyond the "traditional" medical model. Primary-care physicians and allied professionals are called upon more frequently to address parental concerns about developmental delays, poor school performance, or behavioral problems. As a result, pediatricians, family practitioners, pediatric nurses, social workers, and speech/language specialists are faced with the issue of developmental and psychological testing. The degree of the clinician's involvement in testing varies from interpretation of reports to performing screening or assessments. In many cases, the primary health care professional assumes the role of case manager.

Unfortunately, cooperation between disciplines often has been limited because of poor communication, particularly in regard to developmental and psychological testing, where acronyms, statistics, and jargon abound. Even professionals from mental health disciplines such as child psychiatrists or psychiatric social workers sometimes are overwhelmed.

The purpose of this book, therefore, is to provide the clinician with practical information regarding developmental and psychological testing, thereby making the health care professional an "educated consumer." This text does not simply describe how psychologists perform testing; rather, it provides information to help clinicians understand what the tests contain, what their strengths and limitations are, and how they can be incorporated into practice. The book is unique in that rather than simply providing the clinician with a voluminous listing of developmental and psychological tests, it is couched within the framework of addressing two of the most common "new morbidity" problems, namely, suspected developmental delay and difficulties in school performance. Within this framework, selected tests that are used to evaluate different areas of function are discussed in applied terms. Descriptions of the tests, an overview of their strengths and limitations, and suggestions as to how these techniques might be applied to office practice are provided. Related topics such as learning disabilities, attention deficits, language disorders, providing feedback, clinical clues, and diagnostic algorithms are discussed. Care is taken to minimize the amount of detail, and clinical applications and illustrative examples are emphasized. Insight is provided into clinical decision making that is based on developmental and psychological test results.

The text is geared for physicians, allied health professionals, and psychologists who practice in clinical settings. It is hoped that this book will serve as an explanatory reference guide for health care professionals who work with children, enabling these professionals to provide *total* care to their young patients and their families.

GLEN P. AYLWARD

❋ Contents

I. DEVELOPMENTAL ASSESSMENT

APPENDIXES

Practitioner's Guide to Developmental and Psychological Testing

1 ❋ Developmental Assessment

1 ❀ Introduction and Terminology

1.1. INTRODUCTION

The most common concerns in pediatrics and other primary-care specialties are not the same as they were 20 years ago. During the past several decades there has been increased emphasis on "total health care." This societal concern has broadened the role of the primary-care physician, requiring increased involvement with psychological and developmental testing. There is a particular need to be knowledgeable about these evaluation tools because it is estimated that one out of ten children has some type of developmental handicap or a less severe learning problem. Following the enactment of PL 94-142 [Education for All Handicapped Children Act (1975)], about 5% of all school-aged children received special education services for learning disabilities (LDs) despite an estimated 11% to 13% prevalence of LD.

Similarly, the need for early developmental assessment has intensified following the implementation of PL 99-457, the Amendments to the Education for All the Handicapped Act (1986).[1,2] This legislation extended PL 94-142 by mandating, under the Preschool Grant Program, early intervention services for at-risk children ages 3 to 5 years. In addition, the Handicapped Infants and Toddlers Program component (Part H) has provided incentive grants to initiate programs for the birth to 3-year high-risk population. More recently, PL 102-119,[3] the Individuals with Disabilities Education Act Amendments of 1991 (IDEA), reauthorized family-centered programs for infants and toddlers from birth to age 3 (Part H). Specifically, PL 102-119 targets minority, low-income, inner-city, and rural populations. The law mandates improved cooperation between health care and special education disciplines. Consequently, physicians will be integrally involved in the *early* identification of developmental delays and children who are at biological or environmental risk. Primary-care physicians will actively participate in the formulation of "individualized family service plans" (IFSPs) and interpret results of screenings and evaluations to parents. Furthermore, there is an increasing population of high-risk nursery graduates who will be the health care responsibility of primary-care physicians. These children are at increased risk for high-prevalence, low-severity learning problems such as deficits in visual–motor integration, visual perception, reading, language, mathematics, and attention/concentration.[4,5] Pediatricians and other primary-care physicians therefore are faced with two challenges: (1) earlier, more accurate identification of developmental problems and (2) increased need for detection and intervention for later learning difficulties (LDs).

Parents, when confronted with these problems, will typically first contact their child's physician, seeking advice about: (1) the results of previous psychological/developmental testing; (2) the implications of these results on their child's educational program and placement; (3) the need for additional testing and guidance as to what type it should be; and (4) the physician performing the screening or preliminary evaluations in his/her office. Regardless of whether the physician intends to administer tests or prefers to review consultant and/or school reports, he/she should be familiarized with the types of psychological and developmental tests available, basic properties of these tests, some of their common pitfalls,[6,7] which tests are devised for diagnosing particular problems, and ways to extract salient information from psychological reports.

The Committee on Children with Disabilities[8] urges that "The pediatrician should help arrange for confirmatory tests and appropriate pediatric developmental examinations and for the interpretation of test results to the family in a nonthreatening environment" (p. 527). The committee commented further that ". . . the pediatrician should seek a report of the child's actual school and behavioral performance at regular intervals" (p. 527). Unfortunately, despite these strong recommendations, many practitioners feel ill-equipped to meet these critical needs.

Psychological and developmental assessment instruments can be grouped into four general categories: (1) cognitive/developmental; (2) academic/achievement; (3) neuropsychological/perceptual; and (4) emotional/personality. These four areas are not mutually exclusive, and a significant overlap is found.[9] However, merely grouping test instruments in these four categories is neither practical nor useful for the primary-care physician. Familiarization with developmental and psychological testing is best achieved by addressing two of the most common behaviorally oriented referral problems faced by practitioners, namely, suspected developmental delay and impaired school performance.

Similar to the clinical reasoning process used in other areas of pediatrics, decision rules and a differential diagnosis must be entertained in psychological and developmental testing. Administration of the same tests for *all* problems is clinically inappropriate and is not cost-effective. In the algorithm or work-up of a young patient with suspected developmental delay, the differential diagnosis should, in part, include mental retardation, an emerging learning disability, language dysfunction, environmental deprivation, or combinations of these etiologies. Information, therefore, must be obtained from three basic areas: (1) developmental (cognitive/motor), (2) language, and (3) behavioral/adaptive. Similarly, with the child who experiences difficulty in learning or academic achievement, a variety of etiologies should be considered, including mental retardation, LDs, attention-deficit disorders, and/or emotional problems. To define the cause, information is required from five major areas: (1) intelligence (IQ), (2) level of academic achievement, (3) attention/concentration skills, (4) perceptual (visual–motor) function, and (5) behavior.

In summary, counseling and advising parents about developmental delays, educational needs, or the rights of their child is a difficult challenge for professionals at best. It is hoped that this textbook will enhance the ability of practitioners to approach this task in a more knowledgeable and efficient manner, thereby providing an invaluable service both for their young patients and for their families.

1.2. TERMINOLOGY

Developmental and psychological evaluations provide objective measurement of a child's development, behavior, cognitive abilities, or level of achievement. The score obtained usually is compared to standardized, norm-referenced scores, which are derived from a group of similar children. However, no test is without error, and by definition, approximately 5% of the general population obtain, on any particular test, scores that fall outside the range of "normal." Moreover, the range of normal is *descriptive*, not *diagnostic*[10]; it describes problem-free individuals, but it does not diagnose them. Test scores that fall outside the normal range could simply be a chance variation. Pediatricians should be aware that there are three major sources of variation that may significantly affect the outcome of diagnostic testing: (1) reproducibility of a given test, (2) the range of variation among normal children, and (3) the range of variation among children who have compromised functioning.[10]

A basic familiarity is necessary with terms that relate to psychometric issues and test interpretation, regardless of whether the physician chooses to administer these examinations or simply review test data generated by other professionals. Terminology can be divided into three categories: (1) terms used to detect dysfunction in populations, (2) psychometric terminology, and (3) terms used in test interpretation. The definitions that follow are intended to be parsimonious and practical and should prove a useful reference source for the practitioner.

1.2.1. Terminology Used to Detect Dysfunction in Populations

The study of the distribution of diseases in a population is referred to as *epidemiology*. More recently, the definition of epidemiology has been expanded to include the "study of the distribution and determinants of the varying rates of diseases, injuries, or other health states in human populations."[11] Epidemiologic terminology, as applied to developmental and psychological testing, will be reviewed in the text that follows. It should be emphasized that measurement poses a problem in pediatrics and psychology because of an absence of universally accepted "gold standards." This issue will be discussed in greater detail below (Section 1.3).

Sensitivity measures the proportion of children with a specific problem who are positively identified by a test. Children having a disorder but who are not identified by the test are considered "false negatives." Sensitivity is sometimes termed copositivity, if the "gold standard" (the criterion used to determine the presence of a given problem) is not definitive.

Specificity measures the proportion of children who actually are normal and who also are correctly determined by a given test not to have a problem. Children who are normal but who are incorrectly determined by a test to be delayed or learning-disabled are termed "false positives." Specificity is sometimes called conegativity if the "gold standard" is not definitive as to the presence or absence of a disorder. Sensitivity and specificity are presented graphically in Figure 1.1.

Predictive value of a positive test refers to the proportion of children with a positive test result who actually are delayed or learning-disabled. The lower the prevalence of a disorder, the lower will be the positive predictive value. Sensitivity may be a better measure in low-prevalence problems.

Predictive value of a negative test refers to the group of children with a negative test result who indeed do not have developmental delays or disabilities. The value is influenced by the frequency or prevalence of a problem; in low-prevalence problems, specificity may be a better measure.

Prevalence rate refers to the number of children in the population with a given disorder in relation to the total number of children in the population.

Gold Standard (Outcome Measure)

	Delayed (+)	Normal (−)
Delayed (+)	A Children with delays who were picked up by test	B Normal children identified as being delayed by test
Normal (−)	C Children with delays who were not identified on test	D Normal children who also scored 'normal' on test

Test

Sensitivity = A/A + C   Specificity = D/B + D

FIGURE 1.1. Sensitivity and specificity.

Incidence rate indicates the risk of developing a disorder, namely, new cases of a problem that develop over a period of time. The relationship between incidence and prevalence can best be illustrated by the following equation: prevalence rate equals the incidence rate multiplied by the duration of the disorder.

A *Type I error* occurs when, after testing, it is assumed that a difference from normal exists in a child's test scores or developmental levels when, in actuality, there is no difference. A value of $p \leq .05$ means that there is a 5% or less probability of incorrectly determining that a deviance from normal exists (odds are 1 in 20 that the difference would occur by chance alone). This term is equated with level of statistical significance.

A *Type II error* exists when it is assumed that there is no difference in test scores from normal when, in reality, a difference actually is present. This type of error can result from small numbers or chance, and power estimates (described below) enable determination of the probability of a type II error.

Hypothesis testing refers to a series of steps in the decision-making process. The steps typically include the development of a research question, the formulation of a null hypothesis, and the selection of a test statistic that determines whether differences between samples are real or the result of chance.

The Null hypothesis refers to a formal statement indicating that there is *no* difference between two or more groups. For example, there is no difference in IQ between children with attention deficits and children without attention deficits. Typically researchers attempt to disapprove (reject) the null hypothesis.

The *power* of a test refers to the ability of the test to detect a difference between groups when such a difference really exists. In essence, it is the probability of *not* making a type II error.

An excellent resource on measurement issues, data analysis, and how to read the developmental/behavioral literature is found in a special issue of the *Journal of Developmental Behavioral Pediatrics* entitled "Methodological Issues in Developmental and Behavioral Pediatrics."[12]

1.2.2. Psychometric Terminology

The ability to assign numbers to individuals in systematic ways as a means of identifying properties of these individuals is referred to as "measurement." The description, organization, and evaluation of these measurements is psychometric theory.

Reliability refers to consistency or accuracy in measurement. Reliability is concerned with how much error is involved in measurement or how much an obtained score varies from the "true score." One type of reliability, *internal consistency*, suggests that all components of the test are measuring a cohesive construct or set of constructs (e.g., verbal ability, visual–motor skills). Stated differently, all items are highly intercorrelated. *Test–retest reliability* is particularly pertinent in developmental and psychological testing, because it takes into consideration the "true score" and error. This reliability addresses whether the same score would be obtained if a specific test were to be readministered. The length of time between the two administrations of the test is critical in regard to this measurement, i.e., the closer in time the test was readministered, the greater the reliability estimate.

Validity indicates whether a test measures what it purports to measure, i.e., if the items are representative of the domain that supposedly is measured by the test. *Content validity* addresses whether a test covers the material it is presumed to cover. *Criterion-related* validity compares a test score with some external criterion or outcome measure; if this criterion occurs at some future time, the comparison would be termed *predictive validity*. *Construct validity* examines the meaning of a test, namely, the extent to which a test measures a given psychological or developmental trait or construct. Test-related factors (examiner–examinee rapport, handicaps, motivation), criterion-related factors, or intervening events (acute or chronic interfering condition) could affect validity. A specific test can be reliable, yet it may be invalid when used to evaluate a function that it was not designed to measure.[13] Moreover, describing a measure as a "standardized test" does not necessarily mean it is reliable or valid; this simply means the test contains a uniform set of procedures for administration and scoring.

Age equivalent refers to the age at which a child's test score would be considered "average." The age equivalent is computed by obtaining a raw score and comparing it to standardized age norms. The term is often used in developmental assessment; however, it should be considered a relatively gross estimate. Age equivalents routinely are broken down into fractions of years. For example, an age equivalent of 2–11 indicates that the child's performance equals the average performance of the normative group of children aged 2 years, 11 months. This term will be discussed in more detail in Section 5.4 on providing feedback.

Grade equivalent is the grade level at which a child's test score would be considered "average." A grade equivalent is computed by obtaining a raw score and comparing it to standardized grade norms. This estimate is often used in the determination of eligibility for learning disabilities' assistance. A grade equivalent of 4.3 in mathematics means the child's math score was identical to the average score obtained by children in the third month of the fourth grade. Problems with this concept are outlined in Chapter 7.

The *ratio IQ/DQ* is computed as mental age (obtained by the use of a test score) divided by the child's chronologic age, times 100 (MA/CA × 100). IQ/DQ ratio scores are not comparable at different age levels and generally are not used very much in contemporary standardized testing.

Deviation IQ is a method of IQ/DQ estimation that allows for comparability of scores across ages and is used with most major psychological and developmental test instruments. The deviation IQ/DQ is norm-referenced and normally distributed, with the same standard deviation (SD); typically the mean (M) is 100, and the SD is 15 or 16.

1.2.3. Test Interpretation Terminology

Once the sample to be studied has been identified and the tests have been developed and administered, the test results are reported and interpreted. This interpretation includes an array of descriptive terminology, which is highlighted below.

The *normal range* is a statistically defined range of developmental characteristics or test scores that have been established in the absence of detectable delays or disabilities and is measured by a specific method (see Figure 1.2).

The *mean* (M) is the arithmetic average of the total of scores in a distribution. This measure of central tendency can be affected by variations (extreme scores) in the distribution. The mean may therefore be misleading in scores obtained from a highly variable sample (i.e., one with very high or low outlying scores).

The *mode,* a measure of central tendency, is the most frequent or common score in a distribution.

The *median* is defined as the middle score that divides a distribution in half when all the scores have been arranged in order of increasing magnitude. It is the point above and below which 50% of the scores fall; this measure is not affected by extreme scores and therefore would be useful in a highly variable sample (see Figure 1.2).

Range is a measure of variability that reflects the difference between the lowest and highest scores in a distribution. The range does not provide information about data between the two extreme values in the distribution.

Standard deviation (SD) is a measure of variability that indicates the extent to which scores deviate from the mean. The SD is the average of individual deviations from the mean in a specified distribution of test scores. The greater the SD, the more variability is found in test scores (see Figure 1.2).

Standard error of measurement (SEM) estimates the error factor in a test

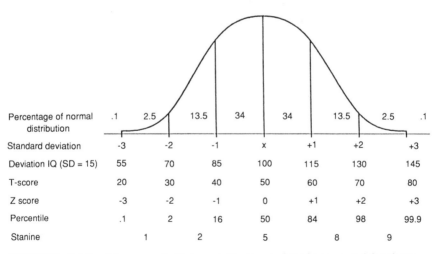

Percentage of normal distribution	.1	2.5	13.5	34	34	13.5	2.5	.1
Standard deviation	-3	-2	-1	x	+1	+2	+3	
Deviation IQ (SD = 15)	55	70	85	100	115	130	145	
T-score	20	30	40	50	60	70	80	
Z score	-3	-2	-1	0	+1	+2	+3	
Percentile	.1	2	16	50	84	98	99.9	
Stanine		1	2	5	8	9		

FIGURE 1.2. Relationships among test interpretation terms, plotted on a normal distribution.

that is the result of sampling or test characteristics, taking into account the M, SD, and size of the sample. The SEM is produced by administering a test, readministering a test, and then calculating how closely the two scores agree. Close scores yield a smaller SEM. In 95% of cases, the interval of approximately two times the standard error of measurement above or below a child's score would contain the "true" score. This would be considered a 95% confidence interval. This concept should always be considered when reviewing or comparing test data. In a 90% confidence interval, an interval of 1.64 times the SEM above and below a child's score would contain the "true" score.

Percentile rank is a derived score that reflects a child's standing within a group. For example, if a child scored at the 75th percentile, he/she would have scored as well as or better than 75% of the children taking that particular test (thereby being in the top 25%) (see Figure 1.2). This score enables the clinician to compare a child's performance to that of peers.

Standard scores specify how many standard units above or below the normative mean a specific child's score falls. The standard score provides a very precise method of pinpointing an individual child's performance in comparison to his/her peers. The standard score describes a child's performance by indicating the number of SDs above or below the mean that child's score is.

Z scores are standard-scale scores with a mean of 0 and a SD of 1. This concept indicates the number of standard deviation units a score falls above or below the mean. A negative Z score indicates that the child performed below average; a positive Z score is indicative of above-average performance (Figure 1.2).

A *T-score* is a standard score based on a distribution having an M of 50 and a SD of 10. Therefore, a T-score of 70 would be two SDs above the mean (see Figure 1.2).

The *stanine* concept is a single-digit scoring system with an M of 5 and a SD of 2. Scores are expressed in whole numbers from 1 to 9 (see Figure 1.2).

The relationship among test interpretation terms is indicated in Figure 1.2. It should be emphasized that the selection of terms is not exhaustive; however, the terms listed above should enable the practitioner to be able to interpret test data in a more accurate fashion.

1.3. EXAMPLES

As was suggested above, sensitivity and specificity are important concepts in developmental and psychological testing. These measures are used to evaluate the predictive accuracy of a test instrument in regard to a child's actual outcome. Outcome routinely is determined by a criterion measure that is considered to be a "gold standard." However, in developmental and psychological testing, so-called gold standards are not as clearcut or universally accepted as are laboratory values; in fact, many tests that are used as gold standards are, in actuality, poor choices. Practitioners therefore must be aware of the reliability, validity, and potential limitations of a test, particularly when the test will be used as the determinant of a child's level of functional development.

Kenny and Holden[13] provide several excellent examples. Many developmental tests such as the Denver Developmental Screening Test (DDST)[14] are designed to span wide age ranges. In the 0- to 2-year age range, the language section of the DDST contains 13 items, five of which measure expressive language. The gross motor scale includes 21 items, the fine motor area, 20. Therefore, success or failure of one language item has a disproportionate influence on overall test results, in comparison to the child's performance on a motor item. Thus, the content validity of the instrument has been compromised by naturally occurring developmental variations (more motor items than language items can be measured at this age).[13] The potential problem in using this measure as a gold standard becomes obvious.

Similarly, with older children the Wechsler Intelligence Scale for Children-Revised (WISC-R)[15] is used to measure intelligence from ages 6 to 17 years. However, as Kenny and Holden[13] suggest, the number of items applicable to children in the 6- to 7-year age range is limited; this produces increased variability and potential inflation of scores in comparison to those obtained by older students. This situation is sometimes referred to as a weak test "floor." At younger ages, success or failure on one or two items would have significant effects on overall test scores. Again, this limitation weakens assumptions that can be made from these test data.

Standardization samples (from which the normative data are derived) also must be comparable to the population to which the test is being applied. This particular issue becomes problematic in the application of a test such as the Bayley Scales of Infant Development (BSID)[16] to populations of handicapped children. Blind children, those with neuromotor impairment (cerebral palsy), or severe language dysfunction require special testing considerations. The issue then is raised as to whether the developmental quotients obtained from these exceptional children are comparable to norms.[17] Clinical samples also should be used by test developers for comparative purposes in these populations.

Finally, descriptive statistics (range, mean, median, mode, and standard deviation) obtained from clinical populations can differ markedly from those derived from the normative sample. The IQ scores in children

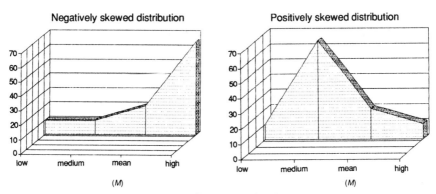

FIGURE 1.3. Differences in distributions.

from indigent populations may be positively skewed (condition in which more children score low) and have more variability (wider spread under the "curve"). Conversely, in pediatric practices primarily comprised of children from upper-socioeconomic-status households, the IQ curve may be negatively skewed (more children score higher), with a corresponding smaller standard deviation. These issues have significant ramifications regarding the clinical interpretation of scores (see Figure 1.3).

In summary, although measurement issues are viewed as tedious or mundane aspects of clinical practice, these issues are, nonetheless, critical. Given that diagnoses, placement decisions, and future expectations are made (rightly or wrongly) based on developmental and psychological test data, awareness of testing and measurement issues is necessary for the practitioner.

REFERENCES

1. DeGraw, C., Edell, D., Ellers, B., et al., 1988, Public Law 99-457: New opportunities to serve young children with special needs, *J. Pediatr.* **113**:971–974.
2. Blackman, J. A., Healy, A., and Ruppert, E. S., 1992, Participation by pediatricians in early intervention: Impetus from Public Law 99-457, *Pediatrics* **89**:98–102.
3. U. S. Congress, 1992, Early intervention program for infants and toddlers with disabilities; Proposed rulemaking, *Fed. Register,* **57**(85):18986–19012.
4. Vohr, B. R., and Garcia-Coll, C. T., 1985, Neurodevelopmental and school performance of very low-birth-weight infants: A seven year longitudinal study, *Pediatrics* **76**:345–350.
5. Eilers, B. L., Desai, N. S., Wilson, M. A., and Cunningham, M. D., 1986, Classroom performance and social factors of children with birth weights of 1250 g or less: Follow-up at 5 to 8 years of age, *Pediatrics* **77**:203–208.
6. Frankenburg, W. K., Chen, J., and Thornton, S. M., 1988, Common pitfalls in the evaluation of developmental screening tests, *J. Pediatr.* **113**:1110–1113.

 7. Aylward, G. P., 1987, Developmental assessment: Caveats and a cry for quality control, *J. Pediatr.* **110:**253–254.
 8. Committee on Children with Disabilities, 1986, Screening for developmental disabilities, *Pediatrics* **78:**526–528.
 9. Aylward, G. P., 1988, Infant and early childhood assessment, in: *Assessment Issues in Child Neuropsychology* (M. G. Tramontana and S. R. Hooper, eds.), Plenum Press, New York, pp. 225–248.
10. Riegelman, R. K., 1981, *Studying a Study and Testing a Test. How to Read the Medical Literature*, Little, Brown, Boston.
11. Duncan, D. F., 1988, *Epidemiology: Basis for Disease Presentation and Health Promotion*, Macmillan, New York.
12. Drotar, D. (ed.), 1991, Methodological issues in developmental and behavioral pediatrics, *J. Dev. Behav. Pediatr.* **12:**1991.
13. Kenny, T. J., Holden, E. W., and Santilli, L., 1991, The meaning of measures: Pitfalls in behavioral and developmental research, *J. Dev. Behav. Pediatr.* **12:**355–360.
14. Frankenburg, W., 1967, Denver Developmental Screening Test, *J. Pediatr.* **71:**181–194.
15. Wechsler, D., 1974, *Manual for the Wechsler Intelligence Scale for Children—Revised*, The Psychological Corporation, New York.
16. Bayley, N., 1969, *Manual for the Bayley Scales of Infant Development*, The Psychological Corporation, New York.
17. Gyurke, J., and Aylward, G. P., 1992, Issues in the use of norm-referenced assessments with at-risk infants. *Child Youth Fam. Serv. Q.* **15:**6–8.

2 ❀ Overview of Evaluation Considerations

2.1. INTRODUCTION

Physicians who provide comprehensive health care for children have frequent contact during the first several years of life with the child and his or her family. This contact affords the potential for early identification of developmental delays. However, only approximately 15% to 30% of pediatricians routinely use developmental screening instruments; frequently these screening inventories are administered to children already suspected of having delays, to confirm that these delays truly exist.[1-3] However, screening instruments do not *confirm* a diagnosis; rather, they establish the need for additional, more in-depth testing. Practitioners must appreciate that development is determined by a complex interaction of multiple factors; screening or assessment methods that do not acknowledge this complexity cannot be considered comprehensive.[4] Moreover, developmental change is supported, facilitated, or impeded by environmental influences.[5]

There is significant confusion regarding the terms "screening," "assessment," and "surveillance."[6,7] *Developmental screening* refers to the process of testing whole populations of children, identifying those at high risk for unsuspected deviations from normal, and referring them for further diagnostic assessment. The goal of screening is to detect children who are developmentally at risk, who otherwise would not be identified (i.e., those with problems such as mild mental retardation, speech or language delays, or subtle motor deficits). Screening should be periodic, brief, inexpensive, valid, and reliable, and should include a broad developmental focus.[4]

Assessment is defined as making an evaluation or estimation of development, the end product being a clinical decision by the examiner as to what intervention would be appropriate to facilitate development. Stated differently, an assessment determines the existence of a delay or disability;

15

it is *conclusive* and is based on data from multiple sources. Formal testing, parent interview, and home observations routinely are utilized in developmental assessment. The end result of an assessment is an individual program plan that occurs after an intervention decision has been made. Therefore, screening procedures are *indicative*, whereas diagnostic assessments are more *definitive*. Screening flags those children who need further assessment. Because of test limitations and developmental issues, both procedures are more accurate in preschoolers than in infants or toddlers. Practitioners should acknowledge the broad spectrum of individual differences in children and realize that a specific range of abnormality is elusive. However, the further away from "average" a child is, the less is the likelihood that he or she is normal.

Surveillance involves the periodic assessment of development in relation to the child as a whole. It is a continuous process in which observations are performed during all child health care encounters.[6,7] Development is viewed in the context of the child's overall well-being, and screening tests may be incorporated into the surveillance process. Surveillance essentially is a monitoring process that includes reviewing developmental milestones with parents, informal use of items selected from various developmental schedules, and reliance upon "clinical judgment."[8] Such judgment, however, must be accurate, and physicians' subjective impressions and clinical judgment often are weak in this regard.[8,9] In fact, Illingworth[9] has emphasized caution in regard to making *spot diagnoses*, where practitioners often are misled either by positive attributes such as the child's charm or cuteness or by negative factors such as unattractive appearance, small size, or physical handicap. Reciprocally, in a recent study on identification and management of psychosocial and developmental problems in primary care,[10] clinicians were reported to have identified developmental problems in 27% of their patients. Recognition of a problem was related to the visit being for well-child versus acute care and if the clinician felt he or she knew the child well.[10] Both of these characteristics obviously pertain to developmental surveillance.

As was indicated previously, in addition to utilizing screening instruments, primary-care physicians may assess development by (1) parental reports of developmental milestones, (2) clinical appraisal during routine medical examinations, (3) observation of specific motor milestones, and (4) observation of speech and language skills.[11] Unfortunately, parental recall of milestones may be unreliable, and clinical appraisals or informal evaluations often are ineffective in detecting mild to moderate delays. Few young children are identified early whose IQs subsequently fall in the moderately deficient to marginal range (IQ 52–83). Moreover, fewer than 50% of children with IQs less than 52 are identified before school age. Many pediatricians rely on the age of attainment of motor milestones to be indicative of developmental delays, although 80% of children with mild mental retardation and 50% of those with moderate mental retardation will display *normal* milestones. Recently it has been reported that the more subtle, so-called "high-prevalence" disabilities (e.g., speech impairment, developmental delay) are typically identified after 3 years of age (only 21% before age 5).[12]

Therefore, in the evaluation of a young patient with suspected developmental delay, the differential diagnosis should include (1) mental retardation, (2) an emerging learning disability, (3) language dysfunction, (4) environmental deprivation, or (5) combinations of these etiologies. In this evaluation, information should be obtained from three areas: (1) developmental (cognitive, motor), (2) language, and (3) behavioral/adaptive. A more detailed description of these three areas and their corresponding test instruments follows in the next several chapters.

One final note regarding the term *developmental delay* deserves mention. With the passage of PL 99-457 (Parts H and 619) and the subsequent Individuals with Disabilities Education Act (IDEA) (see Chapter 1 for further discussion), emphasis has been placed on *noncategorical diagnosis* and *noncategorical service* delivery. *Developmental delay* is recognized as an appropriate "nonclassification" to declare a child's eligibility to receive developmental and family support intervention services.[13] This allows for provision of services, but it circumvents the problem of "labeling" a child.

2.2. DEVELOPMENTAL EVALUATION INSTRUMENTS

There is a plethora of developmental evaluation instruments available for physician use; 15 that are frequently encountered are included in this section. The list is by no means exhaustive; rather, it reflects the clinical bias of this author and the relative probability that the evaluation technique will be encountered by the practitioner. In addition, both screening and more detailed assessment instruments are included in this review. Some of these evaluation instruments can be administered by primary-care physicians, whereas others are traditionally administered by psychologists or other professionals whose clinical training may have different foci. A list of these instruments is found in Table 2.1.

2.2.1. Denver Developmental Screening Test

The Denver Developmental Screening Test[14–16] (DDST) is the most extensively taught and validated screening test used in the United States and other countries. It is estimated that the DDST has been administered

TABLE 2.1. Developmental Evaluation Instruments

Developmental testing instruments	Developmental area assessed					Type		Appropriate for office use		Age range
	Cognitive	Motor	Neurodevelopmental/ Neurological	Language	Adaptive/Behavioral	Screen	Detailed	Yes	No	
Denver Developmental Screening Test (DDST)/Denver II	X	X		X	X	X		X		0–6 years
Prescreening Developmental Questionnaire (R-PDQ)	X	X		X	X	X		X		0–6 years
Bayley Scales of Infant Development (BSID)/Bayley II	X	X		X			X		X	0–30 months
Gesell Developmental Schedules	X	X		X	X		X	X		0–36 months
Bayley Infant Neurodevelopemntal Screen (BINS)	X	X	X	X		X	X	X		3, 6, 9, 12, 18, 24 months
Milani-Comparetti–Gidoni Neurodevelopmental Screening Examination (MCG)	X	X	X			X		X		0–2 years
Battelle Developmental Inventory (BDI)	X	X		X	X	X	X	X[a]		0–8 years
Differential Ability Scales (DAS)	X			X			X		X	2½–17 years, 11 months
McCarthy Scales of Children's Abilities	X	X		X		X	X		X	0–6 years
Cattell	X			X		X	X		X	2–30 months
Fagan Test of Infant Intelligence	X								X	<1 year
Kent Infant Development Scale (KIDS)	X	X		X	X	X		X		≤1 year
Miller Assessment for Preschoolers (MAP)	X	X	X	X			X	X		2.9–6 years
FirstSTEP	X	X	X	X	X[b]	X		X		2.9–6.2 years

[a]Short form.
[b]Optional.

to 20 to 30 million children worldwide. In the development of this particular screening test, a pool of 240 items was extracted from more than a dozen infant developmental tests. From this pool, a final group of 105 items was selected and standardized on a sample of 1036 children; 82% white, 11% Hispanic, and 7% black. Test–retest and interexaminer reliability figures have been acceptable.[14] The DDST is used to evaluate four developmental areas: personal–social (23 items), fine motor (30 items), language (21), and gross motor (31 items). From the screening battery, about 20 to 25 items typically are administered; this requires approximately 10 to 20 min of testing time.

A "delay" should be suspected if a child fails an item that is successfully completed by 90% of younger children. Although the DDST is designed for screening children from birth to age 6 years, it is best administered for children from 3 months to 3 or 4 years of age.

The materials for administering the DDST consist of a test kit, score sheet, and a reference manual. Test materials in the kit include a red yarn pom–pom, box of raisins, rattle, small bottle with a $\frac{5}{8}$-inch opening, bell, tennis ball, pencil, and eight colored cubes.

The DDST had been criticized because of the relatively long time required to administer it routinely and because it did not provide a profile of the child's rate of development. In response to these criticisms, an abbreviated version was developed that included a revised DDST form that more graphically portrayed the child's developmental rate.[17] The abbreviated version is reported to take half the time to administer as the full DDST and requires only 12 age-appropriate items (three from each of the four areas). If any of these 12 items immediately to the left of a child's chronological age line is failed, the full DDST is administered. In a validation study, the "short DDST" identified low scorers on the Stanford–Binet as accurately as did the full DDST.[16] In a later article, 39 key DDST items were identified, which enabled administration of approximately four items at any one age without any decrease in sensitivity. It is suggested that in populations of children from low-socioeconomic-status households, the abbreviated DDST should be administered first, then followed by the full DDST if necessary.

The DDST yields excellent test specificity (93%), but sensitivity has been poor (mean = 0.41)[18]; the resultant false-negative rate is 59%. Basically, the test instrument underrefers by a 2:1 ratio. Language, particularly expressive language and articulation, is a relatively weak area, and neurodevelopmental issues are overlooked. In addition, pediatricians should be aware that long-term prediction is poor, particularly in attempting to predict later normality from an early, normal DDST result.[19] Meisels[18] delineated several other problems: (1) 48/105 (46%) of the items may be passed by report, (2) cut-off criteria (questionable, abnormal) may obscure mild delays, (3) validation studies do not fully assess accuracy in normal or questionable children, and (4) attempting to span the first 6 years may be too broad an undertaking (e.g., less than 8% of the items are applicable at the 4- to 5-year age range).

In summary, the DDST is a conservative test that errs in classifying as "normal" some children who are experiencing developmental delays. Studies of the DDST indicate that there is a 3% to 4% rate of abnormal scores, 7% to 9% questionable, with 5% of children being untestable.[19] This occurs despite an *expected* "not normal" (abnormal plus questionable) rate of 10% to 13%. The DDST appears to be fairly accurate in identifying children whose Bayley Scales of Infant Development (BSID) scores are ≤68, but it is less reliable in specifying those whose scores fall in the 68 to 84 range. Prediction of early school problems is variable, with specificity being much better than sensitivity.[20,21]

Although the authors emphasize that the DDST is a screening test, it is often misused as a *diagnostic* or *IQ* test. In addition, developmental quotients or mental ages are sometimes computed from the DDST. Use of training materials such as the manual workbook, videotapes, and the proficiency test would help minimize the most significant problems of inaccurate administration and interpretation.[22] The DDST can be a useful *screening instrument*, whether it is administered by the physician or trained office staff, only if practitioners are cognizant of its limitations.

2.2.2. Denver II

A revised DDST, the Denver II,[23,24] recently has been made available. The revision was renormed on more than 2000 children. The Denver II contains 125 items, and a screening and a technical manual are provided. This screening test exhibits a mean examiner–observer reliability of 0.99, whereas mean test–retest reliability is 0.90. The major differences between the Denver II and the DDST are (1) an 86% increase in language items, (2) inclusion of two articulation items, (3) a new age scale, (4) a "caution" scoring option, (5) a five-item behavioral scale (typical behavior, compliance, interest in surroundings, fearfulness, attention span), (6) a 22% decrease in the number of reported items, and (7) new training materials[25] (see Figure 2.1).

As mentioned previously, scoring contains a new component, the *caution* option. A "caution" is scored if the child fails or refuses an item where the age line falls on or between the 75th to 90th percentile. A "questionable" Denver II therefore occurs when the child receives one delay and/or two or more "cautions." This screening test places more emphasis on clinical judgment, and preliminary feedback by test users

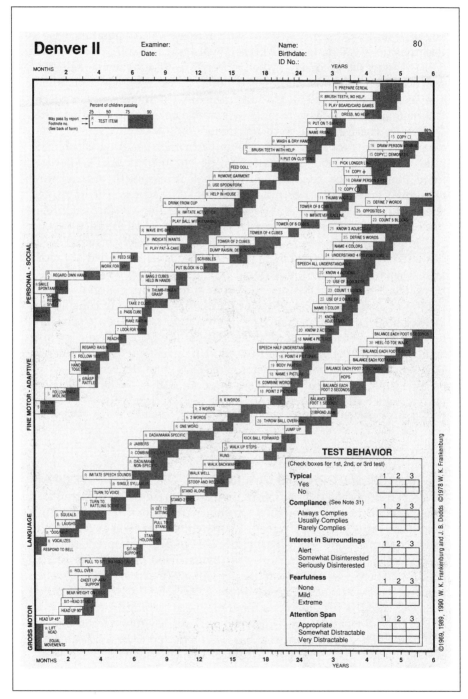

FIGURE 2.1. The Denver II (Copyright Denver Developmental Materials, Inc., reprinted with permission).

suggests improved sensitivity but with a reciprocal potential increase in false positives. Validation data presently are not available.

Recently, the accuracy of the Denver II in developmental screening was evaluated.[26] In this study, 104 children between 3 and 72 months of age were administered individual measures of intelligence, speech–language function, achievement, and adaptive behavior in addition to the Denver II. The Denver II correctly identified 83% of children who had developmental problems (language impairments, learning disabilities, mild mental retardation, or functional developmental delay). However, more than half the children with normal development also received abnormal, questionable, or untestable Denver-II scores. Therefore, test specificity was 43%.[26] Items in the language domain were most helpful in discriminating children with and without developmental difficulties.

In defense of the Denver II, the authors specifically state "It is not designed to yield a Developmental Quotient, nor is it designed to predict later learning disabilities, emotional problems, special education placement, etc. The Denver II is designed simply to identify children who are not 'up to snuff . . .' "[25] (p. 96). Dworkin's (8) suggestion to consider the Denver II as a developmental chart or inventory, rather than a screening test per se, appears very appropriate. Use of the Denver II in a manner similar to a growth chart would be helpful in developmental surveillance. Finally, it seems that major criticisms of the DDST and Denver II should not be directed at the instruments themselves but, rather, to the applications beyond which the instruments originally were designed for.[8,25]

2.2.3. Prescreening Developmental Questionnaire

In 1976, the Prescreening Developmental Questionnaire (PDQ) was developed, incorporating 97 DDST items. These items were formulated into questions to be answered by the child's parent or caretaker.[27] In this brief (5–10 min) first-stage screen, the parent or caretaker is required to answer ten questions about the child related to age-appropriate developmental tasks. The questionnaire was standardized on a sample of 1155 children. There was 68% to 100% agreement (mean = 93%) between parental reports and actual scores on the DDST, and it was estimated that the PDQ could reduce the need for complete screening by 69%. A high school educational level was suggested as necessary for accurate completion of the PDQ, although it also has been reported to be applicable in a predominantly black, depressed socioeconomic population.

The questionnaire was revised in 1987 and redesignated as the R-PDQ.[28] This revision was in response to opinions expressed by many clinicians that the previous ten items were often too easy for children to pass and that parents would not have any idea as to how their child had progressed developmentally. The revision currently includes *all* 105 DDST items, and parents are instructed to answer the R-PDQ items until a total of three "no" responses is obtained. Test–retest reliability (1 week) was 94%, and agreement between parents and teachers was 83%.[28] In the standardization sample of 1434 children, suspect scores were found to vary between settings, ranging from 16% among private pediatric practices to almost 50% in Head Start and urban daycare centers. Four color-coded forms are available: 0 to 9 months, 9 to 24 months, 2 to 4 years, and 4 to 6 years. If no delays are reported, follow-up is not necessary; one delay warrants rescreening with the R-PDQ in 1 month, whereas two or more delays mandate administration of the full DDST or Denver II.

The R-PDQ meets the needs of the two-step approach to evaluating children that was recommended by the American Academy of Pediatrics. The first step consists of parent report and an examination of the child, whereas the second step, which utilizes developmental screening, is recommended if results from the first step are suspect. This instrument can be very useful in an office practice and has been reported to identify 84% of those children who subsequently have obtained "abnormal" DDST classifications.

2.2.4. Bayley Scales of Infant Development

The Bayley Scales of Infant Development[29] (BSID) is probably the best instrument available to assess infant development and has for the most part replaced earlier infant tests such as the Cattell.[30] The BSID is generally administered to children from 2 to 30 months, but it can be used with older, developmentally delayed children (although in the latter circumstances only age equivalents, not developmental indices, can be reported).

The BSID consists of three parts: (1) The Mental Developmental Index (MDI) consisting of 163 items, (2) the Psychomotor Developmental Index (PDI), which contains 81 items, and (3) the Infant Behavior Record (IBR), which provides descriptors of the infant's behaviors. On the MDI and PDI, the mean is 100 (SD = 16); 50 is the lowest MDI or PDI. The MDI was designed to "assess sensory–perceptual acuities, discriminations, and the ability to respond to these; the early acquisition of 'object constancy,' memory, learning, and problem-solving ability; vocalizations and the beginnings of verbal communication; and early evidence of the ability to form generalizations and classifications, which is the basis of abstract thinking"[29] (p. 3). Functions assessed with the MDI include perceptual abilities, object permanence, memory, problem-solving skills, imitative abilities, and early symbolic thinking. The PDI provides evaluation of gross and fine motor development, whereas the IBR includes assessment of social, behavioral, and emotional functioning. Therefore, the BSID is helpful in allowing the clinician to evaluate the child's gross motor, fine motor, personal/social, language, and cognitive/adaptive abilities.

The BSID is based on more than 40 years of research, having originated as the California First Year Mental Scale developed in 1933. The test was initially designed to test children in the Berkeley Growth Study. Subsequently, in the 1950s and 1960s, earlier forms were administered to almost 50,000 8-month-old infants enrolled in the National Collaborative Perinatal Project. The present version was standardized on over 1200 children stratified by gender, race, education, and urban/rural area of residence.

The BSID requires approximately 30 to 45 min to be administered by trained examiners, and, therefore, most primary-care physicians will not give the test. Typically, a parent or caretaker is present during the test administration. Items are arranged in ascending order of difficulty, and the average age and normal range (95%) are printed for each item. For example, the item, "retains two cubes," has an average passing age of 4.7 months and a normal range of 3 to 7 months; the average age of passing "walks alone" is 11.7 months, with a range of 9 to 17 months. Basal and ceiling ages are established, and the number of items passed is summed. These sums (MDI and PDI) are compared to norm-referenced tables for the child's age, and from this, developmental quotients are derived. The normative tables also can be used in a fashion where the total number of MDI or PDI items passed is matched to the age at which that number would yield a developmental index of 100. This would provide the child's developmental age equivalent.

Correlations between the MDI and PDI are greater at younger ages; therefore, early on, children with motor handicaps may score low on both the MDI and PDI but then show improvement on the MDI when these indices diverge. Correlations with later IQ scores are generally low in young children, but they improve from age 24 months onward. However, even early developmental delays are prognostically significant. Experience suggests that suspect motor dysfunction and, occasionally, abnormal motor function tend to improve, whereas "not normal" cognitive function frequently stays the same or worsens.[31] Major shifts in cognitive developmental function, often attributed to the cumulative effects of a nonstimulating environment, frequently occur in the 18- to 24-month age range.[5,31]

The BSID is not a test simply learned from perusal of a manual, and many individuals administering the Bayley do so without being qualified.[17] Although test items are ordered chronologically, clinicians should administer in a consecutive fashion those items containing similar content. Failure to develop adequate rapport with the child, inability to keep the infant sufficiently interested, lack of cooperation, the clinician's determination of the "best possible performance," and the influence of other handicapping conditions can be problematic and invalidate test results. Pediatricians should therefore be cautious when they receive these developmental reports and when interpreting the test results.

The BSID has undergone revision and has been renamed the Bayley II.[33] The test was normed on a stratified, contemporary sample of 1700 children. Concurrent validity studies with the original BSID, DDST, the Differential Ability Scales, and McCarthy Scales (to be discussed subsequently) have also been undertaken. The age range for Bayley II is from 1 to 42 months, allowing for overlap with other tests such as the McCarthy Scales or Wechsler Preschool and Primary Scale of Intelligence—Revised (WPPSI-R) (see Chapter 8). The revised Bayley includes new items measuring information processing and memory and learning, and it allows for a more detailed evaluation of language function. Some items from the original BSID were deleted (e.g., headless doll), whereas others were reordered, based on contemporary developmental norms. The BSID-II is a "power test" in that items are arranged in order of difficulty.

The Behavior Rating Scale of the BSID-II is clinically more useful than its predecessor. Four factors, arousal/attention, orientation/engagement, emotional regulation, and motor quality, are produced. The Mental Developmental Indices (MDI) of the BSID and BSID-II are moderately correlated ($r = 0.62$), with the BSID-II MDI being an average of 12 points lower. Moderate correlations between the two Psychomotor Developmental Indices also were found ($r = 0.63$), with the BSID-II PDI being seven points lower than that of the BSID.[33]

Stated differently, an MDI score of 100 on the BSID would yield a BSID-II MDI in the 88 to 92 range (95% confidence interval). A BSID PDI score of 100 would yield a BSID-II PDI of 88 to 93.

Practitioners should be aware that renorming of the BSID (as well as most developmental and psychological tests) is necessary, because normative data become obsolescent every 10 to 15 years. As a result, the mean score of the earlier version of a given test becomes inflated by as much as five or more points.

2.2.5. Gesell Developmental Schedules

The original Gesell was standardized in the 1920s and 1930s on a sample of 107 children. The examination was popularized as a developmental diagnostic tool in 1941, with Gesell and Amatruda stating that "developmental diagnosis is essentially an appraisal of the maturity of the nervous system with the aid of behavior norms"[34] (p. 15). The most recent revision by Knobloch, Stevens, and Malone[35] was published in 1980 and was entitled the *Manual of Developmental Diagnosis* (for the administration and interpretation of the Revised Gesell and Amatruda Developmental and Neurologic Examination). The age range for this examination is from 1 week to 36 months.

The Gesell is divided into (1) 4-week increments up through 56 weeks, (2) 3-month increments from 15 to 24 months, and (3) 6-month intervals at 30 and 36 months. The authors placed significant emphasis on "key" ages, namely, ages at which major developmental acquisitions occur. These ages are: 4, 16, 28, 40, and 52 weeks and 18, 24, and 36 months. Five areas of development are evaluated at each age and include from one to 12 items for each age. These areas are:

1. *Adaptive.* This realm of development is considered the most important and is assumed to be the forerunner of later intelligence. Sensorimotor behaviors, eye–hand coordination, problem-solving, and simple reasoning skills are evaluated. Examples of items that are included in this area are visual following, placing cubes in a cup, performance on formboards, paper-and-pencil imitation, and stacking blocks. There is considerable overlap between this area and the fine motor realm.
2. *Gross motor.* Skills evaluated in this area include postural reactions, head balance, sitting, standing, creeping, and walking. Sample items include pivoting when prone, cruising, running, jumping, and ascending stairs.
3. *Fine motor.* This area involves the use of the hands and fingers in manipulating objects. Sample items consist of holding onto objects, pellet grasp, throwing a ball, stacking cubes, and performance on a pegboard.
4. *Language.* This realm of behavior involves verbal and nonverbal communication such as production of vowel sounds, chuckles, imitation of sounds, word production, comprehension of "no–no," and vocabulary.
5. *Personal–social.* The personal–social area involves the child's reactions to persons and social situations. Sample items include social smile, play behaviors (solo and cooperative), response to mirror, and feeding and dressing skills.

A developmental quotient (DQ) is computed for each area utilizing the formula: maturity age level/chronologic age $\times$ 100 = DQ (see Chapter 1).

A DQ ≤75 is considered abnormal, between 76 and 85 questionable, and ≥86 normal.

In addition, there is a Revised Developmental Screening Inventory[35] in which only two or three items from the Gesell are administered in each of the five developmental areas. Item selection was based on 50% of the children passing a given item at the specified age. Whereas good interrater reliability is reported, validity is less impressive[36] and no standardization is reported.

Directions for the Gesell are relatively brief and subjective, and normative sample sizes have been small. Physicians typically administer this inventory, whereas psychologists do not. An attractive feature of the Gesell is that it yields an estimate of weeks of functioning in each of the five areas and thereby can provide qualitative descriptions of a child's behaviors.

2.2.6. Bayley Infant Neurodevelopmental Screen

The Bayley Infant Neurodevelopmental Screen[37] (BINS) is designed to assess the neuropsychological development of infants from 3 through 24 months of age (corrected for prematurity). The BINS is based on the Early Neuropsychologic Optimality Rating Scales (ENORS),[38–40] and it enables assessment of movement, posture, tone, and developmental delays. A combination of items, extracted from existing tests and techniques and based on a conceptual framework, was used. In actuality, the BINS bridges the concepts of screening and assessment. Although it takes only approximately 10 to 15 min to administer, the BINS should prove highly useful in the prediction of subsequent developmental delays.[41,42] Therefore, the BINS is best considered as a *brief assessment*. The BINS is designed to provide a more thorough assessment than most screening tests by covering functions that would ordinarily be missed with the administration of a developmental or neurological examination in isolation.

There are six BINS versions: 3, 6, 9, 12, 18, and 24 months (Rasch analysis enables testing at ages falling in between these "key" ages), with each version containing 11 to 13 items. Items are grouped into five categories or item clusters: (1) basic neurological function/intactness, (2) receptive functions, (3) expressive functions, (4) processing, and (5) mental activity. The item clusters and examples of component item names for all six preliminary BINS versions are found in Table 2.2.

The BINS contains neurological (reflexes, tone), neurodevelopmental (movement, symmetry), and developmental (object permanence, imitation, language) items, many of which are familiar to the pediatrician. A major premise of the BINS is that it *quantifies* the *qualitative* impressions

TABLE 2.2. Item Clusters and Components Found in the Bayley Infant Neurodevelopmental Screen Standardization Version

			Age (months)			
	3	6	9	12	18	24
I. Basic neurological function/ intactness^a						
1. Primitive reflexes^b	X	X	X	X		
2. Asymmetries	X	X	X	X		
3. Head control	X	X	X	X	X	
4. Muscle tone	X	X	X	X		
5. Abnormal indicators	X	X	X	X		
6. Protective reactions		X	X	X		
7. Drooling/motor overflow					X	X
II. Receptive functions						
1. Auditory	X	X	X	X		
2. Visual	X	X	X	X	X	X
3. Visual tracking	X	X				
4. Verbal receptive			X	X	X	X
5. Understands body parts					X	X
III. Expressive functions						
A. Fine motor/oral motor						
1. Reaching behavior	X	X				
2. Hands open/midline behaviors	X	X	X	X	X	
3. Prehension skills		X	X	X	X	
4. Eye–hand coordination		X	X	X	X	
5. Fine motor control					X	X
6. Vocalizations/verbalizations	X	X	X	X	X	X
7. Names objects/pictures						X
B. Gross motor						
1. Elevates self prone	X					
2. Supports weight	X					
3. Coordinated movement	X	X	X	X		
4. Sitting/rolls over		X	X			
5. Crawling/preambulation			X			
6. Ambulation				X	X	X
7. Throwing/kicking					X	X
8. Ascends stairs					X	X
9. Jumps						X
IV. Processing						
1. Social smile	X					
2. Regards objects	X					
3. Object permanence		X	X	X	X	X
4. Imitative abilities		X	X	X	X	
5. Problem solving		X	X	X	X	X
6. Form boards						X

(*Continued*)

TABLE 2.2. (*Continued*)

	Age (months)					
	3	6	9	12	18	24
V. Mental activity						
1. Goal-directed behaviors	X	X	X	X	X	X
2. Attentiveness	X	X	X	X	X	X
3. Activity level	X	X	X	X	X	X
4. Persistent crying/irritability	X					

[a]Item cluster.
[b]Component item.

gained in the evaluation of an infant or toddler. Scoring is based on Prechtl's *optimality concept*,[43] in which items are scored "optimal" or "nonoptimal" based on specific criteria and then are summed. A percentage score [number optimal/(number optimal + number nonoptimal)] is then calculated. Final cut-off scores are not available at this time because the BINS is currently undergoing national standardization with data from samples of 600 " normals" and 300 "clinical" cases (preterm, SGA, drug-exposed infants, and those with intraventricular hemorrhage, seizures, asphyxia, etc.) currently being collected. Nonetheless, with earlier versions of the ENORS, cutoff scores of 75 to 85% optimal for the 6-, 9-, 12-, and 18-month versions and 65% at 24 months produced the best sensitivity and specificity figures in regard to 36-month outcome (see Table 2.3).

The BINS is geared toward physicians, psychologists, occupational and physical therapists, child-development specialists, and other professionals. By combining a variety of techniques to provide a more comprehensive and inclusive assessment, the BINS can be used to predict the outcome of infants who are at risk. Therefore, the test instrument will be especially useful in developmental follow-up clinics. The pattern or "profile" of scores also is clinically useful. For example, optimal processing (appreciation of object permanence, imitative abilities, problem-solving skills) and mental activity functions (attentiveness to procedures, average activity level, no persistent crying) found in conjunction with either nonoptimal basic neurological function/intactness or gross motor expressive functions would yield a more optimistic prediction than would the reverse. Differentiation of neuromuscular dysfunction from static brain damage is also possible.

It is anticipated that the BINS will be available in the Fall of 1994.

TABLE 2.3. Sensitivity and Specificity Values for the Early
Neuropsychological Optimality Rating Scales (ENORS)

ENORS version	n	Number of items	Correlations with BSID (r)	Sensitivity/ specificity	Cut-off score
3	50	20	0.55–0.61	N/A	N/A
6	520	21	0.80–0.82	82/73	80%
9	504	22	—	76/50	75/80%
12	363	22	0.79–0.83	68/94	85%
18	447	16	—	75/64	80%
24	245	16	0.75–0.82	92/76	65%

2.2.7. Milani-Comparetti–Gidoni Neurodevelopmental Screening Examination

The Milani-Comparetti–Gidoni[44,45] (MCG) is a highly useful technique for the assessment of neuromotor function from birth to 24 months. The MCG, which contains 27 items, is relatively simple, fairly well standardized, and takes approximately 5 min. A very attractive feature of this neurodevelopmental screening instrument is that it can be used in conjunction with a physical examination, and it yields age equivalents.[46,47] The MCG is typically administered by physical therapists, occupational therapists, pediatric neurologists, and developmental pediatricians. The emphasis is on acquisition of motor skills during infancy and elimination or suppression of earlier, more primitive motor patterns. The role of acquisition of new motor skills in development is obvious; reciprocally, certain reflexes must be suppressed so as to allow for the emergence of more sophisticated motor behavior. For example, the foot grasp must be eliminated before a child can stand erect with support; continued presence of the asymmetric tonic neck posture precludes appropriate midline, eye–hand activities.

On the MCG, motor function is divided into spontaneous behavior (nine items) and evoked responses (18 items). The former includes postural control of the body and head (head control when vertical, prone, supine, sitting, standing) as well as active movement (standing up and locomotion). Evoked responses include primitive reflexes (tonic neck, Moro, grasps) as well as righting, parachute (downwards, forwards, sideways, backwards), and tilting reactions. Approximately two-thirds of the items require direct handling, depending on the child's age at testing. A chart is provided[45,47] that allows the clinician to determine the appropriate ages for appearance or elimination of motor behaviors and reflexes. For example, by 4 months, development of head control should be at a stage whereby the head is maintained perpendicular to the ground when the child is held vertically; by 5 months, the head should lean forward when the child is pulled to sit. In reference to evoked responses, the asymmetric tonic neck posture and the Moro response should disappear by 4 months, the palmar grasp by 3.5 months, and the plantar grasp by age 9 months. The downward parachute should be present by 4 months, sideways parachute by 6 months, and forward by 7 months. The vertical lines on the MCG chart[45,47] afford easy assessment of whether the child's motor development is in line with his/her chronological age. The authors suggest that motor retardation associated with mental deficiency usually appears as a general, homogeneous shift toward the left of the age line, whereas a scattering of findings is more likely indicative of specific motor dysfunction such as cerebral palsy.[45]

This test is more of a clinical than a research tool, although there have been further efforts to quantify the data for research purposes.[46,48] Interobserver agreement ranges between 79% and 98%. Active movement and postural control items have the highest level of agreement; equilibrium items (e.g., standing equilibrium) have the lowest. Test–retest agreement ranges between 80% and 100%.[48] It is suggested that the spontaneous behavior, primitive reflexes, and parachute (protective) reaction components be incorporated into the pediatrician's physical examination or during administration of the Denver so as to provide a more thorough measurement of motor function. The test is particularly useful during the first year.[48]

2.2.8. Battelle Developmental Inventory

The Battelle[49] (BDI) is an individually administered assessment instrument that was normed on 800 children. The child's development is evaluated in five areas, from birth to 8 years. These domains include: personal–social, adaptive, motor, communication, and cognitive. The full BDI contains 341 items; the Screening Test consists of 96 items. The inventory was developed utilizing a milestone approach, from which a child's development could be characterized by the attainment of critical skills and/or behaviors in a particular sequence.[50] Item sequences were determined based on the age level at which approximately 75% of the children received full credit for the item (therefore, the number of items at each level is not equal).

The test items are arranged in ten age categories, grouped in 6-month increments from birth to age 2 years and yearly thereafter. Information can be obtained through interview with caregivers, observation in natural settings, or structured assessment (however, agreement between observations and ratings often is modest at best). Items are scored on a three-point system: the child receives a "2" if the response met specified criteria, a "1" if the child attempted the task but was not totally successful (an "emerging" response), or a "0" when the response was clearly incorrect or absent. Domain and subdomain scores have a mean of 10 (SD = 3); the Developmental Quotient (DQ), based on a composite of the five separate domains, has a M of 100 (SD = 15). Age equivalents for domain scores and the Five Motor, Receptive, and Expressive Communication domains are available. Practitioners should consider a 95% confidence interval for the DQ to be ± 8.

Administration of the BDI takes approximately 1 to 2 hr, depending on the child's age; the Screening Test takes 10 to 30 min, again depending on age. The Screening Test should not be administered to children younger than 6 months of age.[50] Computer scoring is available.

The five domains included in the Battelle Developmental Inventory are:

1. *Personal–Social*. This area contains 85 items, grouped into six subdomains: (1) Adult interaction, (2) Expression of feelings/affect, (3) Self-concept, (4) Peer interaction, (5) Coping, and (6) Social role. (Sample items are included in Table 2.4.)
2. *Adaptive*. This domain consists of 59 items, organized into five subdomains: (1) Attention, (2) Eating, (3) Dressing, (4) Personal responsibility, and (5) Toileting (see Table 2.4).
3. *Motor*. The motor domain contains 82 items, clustered into five subdomains: (1) Muscle control, (2) Body coordination, (3) Locomotion, (4) Fine muscle, and (5) Perceptual motor (see Table 2.4).
4. *Communication*. This realm of development includes 59 items, grouped into two subdomains: (1) Receptive communication and (2) Expressive communication (see Table 2.4).
5. *Cognitive*. The cognitive sphere involves 56 items, grouped into four subdomains: (1) Perceptual discrimination, (2) Memory, (3) Reasoning and academic skills, and (4) Conceptual development (see Table 2.4).

A major strength of the BDI is that standardized adaptations for testing handicapped children are provided, including both general and specific alternative administration procedures and scoring criteria. These alternations involve demonstrations of tasks to be performed, specific positioning suggestions, and/or alternative testing materials. This aspect is very helpful in testing motor-, visual-, hearing-, or speech-impaired

TABLE 2.4. Sample Items from the Battelle
Developmental Inventory[a]

Personal/social domain	Communication domain
Plays peek-a-boo	Uses ten or more words
Imitates	Understands prepositions
Describes feelings	Uses plurals
Aware of gender differences	Cognitive domain
Adaptive domain	Finds hidden toy
Uses utensils	Matches geometric forms
Dresses/undresses	Identifies big and small
Dry at night	
Motor domain	
Prehension skills	
Ascends stairs	
Turns doorknob	

[a]From Newborg et al. (49).

children, as well as children with multiple handicaps. The five domains and 24 subdomains enable identification of the child's strengths and weaknesses and help to differentiate overall, versus specific, deficits (e.g., motor). The BDI appears very useful in meeting the PL 99-457 (now PL 102-119) mandate, because the profile enables identification and planning of possible intervention strategies. It also allows for pre- and postintervention testing, and results can be incorporated into the child's Individual Education Program (IEP). Parental involvement, a major component of PL 99-457, is also facilitated as a result of the interview component and accumulation of parental report data.

The BDI correlates well with the BSID ($r = 0.74$ to 0.93), the Peabody Picture Vocabulary Test (Chapter 3), and the Vineland Social Maturity Scale (Chapter 4).[50,51] Pediatricians can anticipate encountering this test instrument with increasing frequency, as several states have selected this instrument for their PL 99-457 (PL 101-119) evaluation programs.

The 96-item Screening Test is more useful for practitioners and consists of two items per age level for each of the five domains. Twenty items each from the Personal–Social, Adaptive, and Motor domains and 18 items each from the Communication and Cognitive domains are included. Approximately 30 items, taking 10 to 30 min, are administered in a typical screening; screening scores are reported to correlate 0.92 to 0.96 with the full BDI.[50]

Recently, criticism has been raised regarding inadequate ceilings and floors for domain scores of the BDI Screening Test.[52] Cut-off scores are provided, with a cut-off score of 1 SD below average indicating borderline performance. Unfortunately, based on these scores, *screening* decisions are referred to as *placement* decisions in the manual. Moreover, for many age levels and domains, one or two raw score points separate a performance of -1 SD from -2.33 SDs; for 46% of the age levels, the range of raw scores that differentiates severely discrepant performance (-2.33 SDs) from a borderline score (-1 SD) was from 0 to 2 points.[52] Therefore, the number of items separating extreme from marginal, or even average, performances is very small or nonexistent. In addition, the difference in scores that are found for children whose birthdays are at the borderline limits of the age intervals can alter interpretation of a child's performance to a significant degree.[53,54] These issues should be considered by clinicians who utilize the BDI Screening Test or review data obtained with the test instrument.

2.2.9. Differential Ability Scales

The Differential Ability Scales (DAS), normed on 3500 children, is a relatively new assessment technique, applicable from age 2 years 6 months to 17 years 11 months. The DAS is particularly useful in the late toddler and early childhood range. The DAS was derived from the earlier (1979) British Ability Scales and is an individually administered profile test that yields a range of developed abilities (not an IQ score). The test instrument takes 25 to 65 min to administer, depending on the child's age. On the DAS, a composite score based on reasoning and conceptual abilities is derived: the General Conceptual Ability Score (GCA) (M = 100, SD = 15, range 45–165). Subtest ability scores have a mean of 50 (SD = 10, range 20–80). In addition to the GCA, Verbal Ability and Nonverbal Ability Cluster Scores are obtained for upper preschool children, whereas Verbal Ability, Nonverbal Reasoning Ability, and Spatial Ability Cluster Scores are produced for the school-age level. Therefore, three levels of interpretation are available: the GCA, cluster scores, and subtest scores (see Figure 2.2). The test is unique in that it incorporates a developmental and an educational perspective.[56]

The DAS contains 17 cognitive and three achievement subtests, grouped in two overlapping levels: preschool and school-age. Twelve core subtests contribute to the General Conceptual Ability Score (GCA), and five additional diagnostic subtests measure short-term memory, perceptual skills, and speed of information processing. The number of subtests that are administered varies, depending on age.

In the $2\frac{1}{2}$ to $3\frac{1}{2}$ year age range, the GCA score is composed of four core subtests; and $3\frac{1}{2}$ years to 5 years 11 months, six subtests are included (see Table 2.5).

In the former age range, the GCA Composite Score includes: (1) block building (perceptual motor task requiring reproduction of two- and three-

AGES AT WHICH EACH SUBTEST IS NORMED

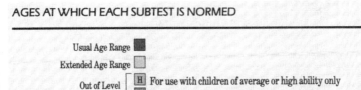

Usual Age Range ■
Extended Age Range ▢
Out of Level
- H For use with children of average or high ability only
- L For use with children of average or low ability only

CORE SUBTESTS	2:6–2:11	3:0–3:5	3:6–3:11	4:0–4:5	4:6–4:11	5	6	7	8
Block Building									
Verbal Comprehension	GCA						L		
Picture Similarities				GCA			L		
Naming Vocabulary									L
Pattern Construction		H							
Early Number Concepts	H						L		
Copying									
DIAGNOSTIC SUBTESTS									
Matching Letter-Like Forms				H			L		
Recall of Digits	H								
Recall of Objects									
Recognition of Pictures	H								L
	2:6–2:11	3:0–3:5	3:6–3:11	4:0–4:5	4:6–4:11	5	6	7	8

Note on Terms: Usual, Extended, Out-of-Level

The terms *usual* and *extended* both indicate that a subtest is appropriate for the full range of ability at that age. The term *out-of-level* means that a subtest is appropriate for **most but not all** children. The subtest either is too easy for children of high ability and should be used only with children of average to low ability (marked "L" in the figure above), or the subtest is too difficult for children of low ability and should be used only with children of average to high ability (marked "H"). See the **Manual** for further discussion of selecting subtests for out-of-level use.

FIGURE 2.2. Cover sheet of the Differential Ability Scales (DAS). From the Differential Ability Scales. (Copyright 1983 by Colin D. Elliott. U.S. adaptation copyright 1990 by The Psychological Corporation. Reproduced by permission. All rights reserved.)

TABLE 2.5. Core and Diagnostic Subtests
of the Differential Ability Scales

Age	Core	Diagnostic
2–6 to 3–5	Block Building	Recall of Digits
	Picture Similarities	Recognition of Pictures
	Naming Vocabulary	
	Verbal Comprehension	
3–6 to 5–11	Copying	
	Pattern Construction	Block Building
	Picture Similarities	Matching Letter-like Forms
	Naming Vocabulary	Recall of Digits
	Verbal Comprehension	Recall of Objects
	Early Number Concepts	Recognition of Pictures

dimensional designs with blocks); (2) verbal comprehension (receptive verbal task necessitating pointing to pictures, following directions); (3) picture similarities (nonverbal reasoning task requiring matching pictures, recognizing relationships based on concepts), and (4) naming vocabulary (verbal expressive task that involves naming objects and pictures of objects). Two diagnostic subtests are also involved in the 2- to 3-year age range: recall of digits (short-term auditory memory) and recognition of pictures (short-term visual memory). From 3 years to 5 years 11 months, early number concepts (nonverbal and verbal knowledge), copying (perceptual motor ability), and pattern construction (spatial reasoning) are included.

The DAS enables identification of a child's capabilities and contains a progressive refinement of abilities as the child's age advances (e.g., from ages 3½ to 5 years 11 months, cluster scores for verbal and nonverbal abilities are produced; at later ages a spatial ability cluster also is included).[57] Each subtest is homogeneous and therefore can be interpreted in terms of content. This interpretability facilitates the identification of the child's specific strengths and weaknesses which is particularly helpful in formulation of intervention strategies. It also offers the capability to "tailor" content to the child's ability level in order to obtain maximum test accuracy while still providing normative interpretation even for out-of-level testing.[57] The General Conceptual Ability Score at 3 years correlates well ($r = 0.76$) with the McCarthy Scales of Children's Abilities (see Section 2.2.10) and the Peabody Picture Vocabulary Test-Revised ($r = 0.84$; see Chapter 3). Overall, the DAS composite scores and GCA correlate with the Wechsler Preschool and Primary Scale of Intelligence-Revised ($r = 0.72$–0.89), Stanford–Binet Intelligence Scale IV ($r = 0.69$–0.77), and the Kaufman Assessment Battery for Children (r = 0.63–0.68). "Out-of-level" testing and extended norms can be used with exceptional children (i.e., bright younger children or older, less able ones). Similar to the BDI, physicians can anticipate encountering the DAS more frequently, as its unique diagnostic potential becomes recognized. The DAS is particularly useful in the evaluation of young ($3\frac{1}{2}$- to 6-year-old) children suspected of having developmental delays, children with hearing or language difficulties, or school-aged students with learning disabilities or mild mental retardation.

2.2.10. McCarthy Scales of Children's Abilities

Some clinicians may question viewing the McCarthy Scales of Children's Abilities[58] (MSCA) as a "developmental" test per se. However, the term IQ was avoided initially, with the test considered to measure the child's ability to integrate accumulated knowledge and adapt it to the tasks of the scales. The test "bridges" the ages where truly developmental tests and those measuring IQ are administered. The MSCA incorporates developmental theory, and its subtests are predictive of skills that are necessary for later school success. Tasks are interesting and attractive for young children, and they are presented in a "rapport-establishing" sequence (see Figure 2.3).

The test is well standardized and psychometrically sound, having been normed on 1032 children. Although the age range is from $2\frac{1}{2}$ to $8\frac{1}{2}$ years, the MSCA is most useful in the 3- to 5-year age range. A total of 18 tests is involved, divided into five categories: verbal (five tests), perceptual–performance (seven tests), quantitative (three tests), motor (five tests), and memory (four tests). Several tests are found on two scales, e.g., the verbal memory task, in which the child is required to memorize series of words or sentences, is found on both the verbal and memory scales (Table 2.6).

The verbal, perceptual–performance, and quantitative scales are combined to yield a General Cognitive Index (GCI) that is sometimes equated with an IQ score. The mean GCI is 100, SD = 16; the mean scale standard score (T-score) for each of the five scales is 50, SD = 10. Fifty is the lowest GCI score, and mental ages and percentiles are provided. Some subtests generate more variance and therefore have been differentially weighted as an adjustment. One of the strengths of the MSCA is that a profile of functioning (with age equivalents) can be obtained in addition to an overall measure of cognitive functioning. Very few IQ tests provide an

McCARTHY SCALES OF CHILDREN'S ABILITIES

Record Form

NAME ____________ AGE ______ SEX ______

HOME ADDRESS ____________

NAMES OF PARENTS OR GUARDIAN ____________

SCHOOL ____________ GRADE ______

PLACE OF TESTING ____________ TESTED BY ____________

REFERRED BY ____________

MSCA PROFILE

Enter the 6 Scale Indexes on the appropriate lines below. Then circle the mark representing the Index for each Scale. Draw a line connecting the circles. Note that the values for GC are different from those for the other Scales.

	Verbal	Perceptual-Performance	Quantitative	General Cognitive	Memory	Motor
SCALE INDEX	______	______	______	______	______	______

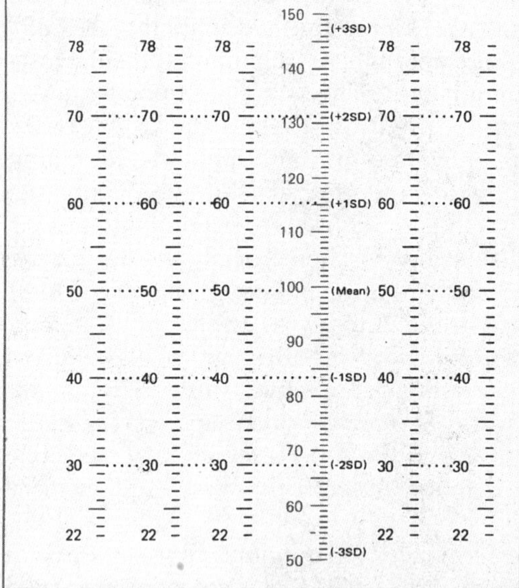

150
(+3SD)
78 78 78 78 78
140
70 70 70 70 70
130 (+2SD)
120
60 60 60 60 60
(+1SD)
110
50 50 50 50 50
100 (Mean)
90
40 40 40 40 40
(-1SD)
80
70
30 30 30 30 30
(-2SD)
60
22 22 22 22 22
50 (-3SD)

	Year	Month	Day
Date Tested	____	____	____
Date of Birth	____	____	____
Age	____	____	____

COMPOSITE RAW SCORES AND SCALE INDEXES

Enter the composite raw scores from the back cover. *Obtain the composite raw score for GC by adding V+P+Q.* Determine the corresponding Scale Indexes from Table 16. (See page 151 of manual for detailed directions.)

Scale	Composite Raw Score	Scale Index
Verbal (V)	______	______
Perceptual-Performance (P)	______	______
Quantitative (Q)	______	______
General Cognitive: Add composite raw scores V+P+Q	______	______ GCI
Memory (Mem)	______	______
Motor (Mot)	______	______

LATERALITY

(Enter information from Laterality Summary on page 5.)

Hand ____________

Eye ____________

THE PSYCHOLOGICAL CORPORATION®
HARCOURT BRACE JOVANOVICH, INC.

76-152AS 9-188731

FIGURE 2.3. Cover sheet of the McCarthy Scales of Children's Abilities (MSCA). From the McCarthy Scales of Children's Abilities. (Copyright 1970, 1972 by The Psychological Corporation. Reproduced by permission. All rights reserved.)

TABLE 2.6. Overview: McCarthy Scales of Children's Abilities

Test	Description	Verbal	Percept/Perf	Quant.	GCI	Memory	Motor
Block building	Copies block structures		X		X		
Puzzle solving	Assembles cut-up pictures		X		X		
Pictorial memory	Recalls pictures shown for 10 sec	X			X	X	
Word knowledge	Identifies pictures/defines words	X			X		
Number questions	Answers number information/basic computational questions			X	X		
Tapping sequence	Copies sequences of notes on xylophone		X		X	X	
Verbal memory	Repeats words, sentences, parts of story	X			X	X	
Right–left orientation	(5 and above) Shows knowledge of R/L		X		X		
Leg coordination	Gross motor tasks of lower extremities						X
Arm coordination	Gross motor tasks of upper extremities						X
Imitative action	Copies simple motor movements						X
Draw-a-design	Copies designs (paper and pencil)		X		X		X
Draw-a-child	Draws rendition of child		X		X		X
Numerical memory	Repeats digits, forward and reverse			X	X	X	
Verbal fluency	Names as many articles as possible in 20 sec from given categories	X			X		
Counting and sorting	Counts and sorts blocks			X	X		
Opposite analogies	Provides opposites to complete sentences	X			X		
Conceptual grouping	Classifies based on color, shape, or size		X		X		

adequate evaluation of both gross and fine motor functioning (although the clinician should consider that the motor scale has the lowest intercorrelation with other MSCA scales). The test takes approximately 45 min in the 3- to 5-year range and is typically administered by psychologists.

The Verbal Scale is considered a measurement of a child's ability to understand, process, and express verbal information. Tests incorporated in this scale evaluate areas such as (1) short-term auditory and visual memory, (2) receptive and expressive word knowledge, (3) short-term auditory memory for words, sentences, or salient components of a short passage read to the child, (4) verbal fluency, (5) verbal abstract concept-formation skills, and (6) verbal labeling (Table 2.6). The Verbal Scale has a limited floor for the youngest age level (up to $3\frac{1}{2}$ years of age), meaning that many of the items simply are too difficult for very young children.[59]

The Perceptual–Performance Scale measures visual–motor coordination and nonverbal practical reasoning abilities. Subtests evaluate: (1) visual–motor/fine motor coordination and visual perception with block building, puzzle-solving, and paper-and-pencil skills; (2) short-term visual memory; (3) right–left orientation; (4) conceptual grouping abilities; (5) spatial skills; and (6) attention to detail. The Quantitative Scale evaluates the child's understanding of numbers, number concepts, and counting, with tasks including answering number questions, short-term auditory memory for digits, and counting and sorting blocks. The Memory Scale contains four subtests that were included in previous scales and measures both auditory and visual short-term memory. Memory can be for meaningful and non-meaningful verbal stimuli as well as for sequential and nonsequential information.[59] Gross and fine motor coordination are measured on the Motor Scale, the former including both leg and arm coordination.

Many subtests (e.g., block building, right–left orientation, leg coordination) have weak test ceilings after age 4 or so.[59] This means that at older ages most children will reach the maximum score, thereby limiting the test's discriminative ability. Reciprocally, many subtests (e.g., puzzle solving, tapping sequence, arm coordination, opposite analogies) are very difficult for $2\frac{1}{2}$- to $3\frac{1}{2}$-year-olds and therefore have a weak test floor.[59]

There are also short forms of the MSCA: the McCarthy Screening Test[58] and Kaufman's Short Form.[61] The latter has been considered more useful[60] and includes six subtests: puzzle solving, word knowledge, numerical memory, verbal fluency, counting and sorting, and conceptual grouping (two subtests each from the Verbal, Perceptual–Performance, and Quantitative Scales). These short forms apparently are not as useful in the youngest age range ($2\frac{1}{2}$–$3\frac{1}{2}$ years).

Physicians should consider a ±8-point 95% confidence interval whenever reviewing the McCarthy GCI. A 10- to 15-point difference in scaled scores between the five scales should be considered significant. In addition, gifted children will score an average of 10 points less on the MSCA than on the Stanford–Binet or Wechsler Intelligence Scale for Children—Revised. Mentally retarded children score approximately 15 to 20 points lower, and the minimum score of 50 may obscure more refined determination of cognitive deficiencies. Children with learning disabilities typically score 8 to 15 points lower on the MSCA than on other tests. Correlations between the MSCA and other tests (Stanford–Binet, WISC-R, Wechsler Preschool, and Primary Scale of Intelligence) range from 0.41 to 0.91. The most recent summary correlation between the GCI and various IQs was $r = 0.74$.[60] The MSCA may not be appropriate for $2\frac{1}{2}$- or 3-year-olds who are below average because the earlier tasks are too hard.

The MSCA has been criticized because of a lack of social comprehension items and because it contains few judgment tasks or abstract problem-solving activities. However, these types of items often are culturally biased. Pediatricians should be aware that the MSCA General Cognitive Index is not readily interchangeable with other intelligence test IQ scores. Because of ceiling issues and the availability of other tests, the MSCA probably should not be used with school-aged children. Finally, the normative data are 20 years old, raising the possibility that they are outmoded. A revision of the MSCA currently is being considered.

2.2.11. Cattell Infant Intelligence Scale

Brief mention of the Cattell Infant Intelligence Scale[30] is warranted, as primary-care physicians may, on occasion, be presented with developmental information derived from this test. It is not considered to be the most appropriate test of infant development, particularly in comparison to the Bayley or Bayley II. The Cattell was developed in 1940 using a standardization sample of 274 children tested at 3, 6, 9, 12, 18, 24, 30, and 36 months. Therefore, item placements at 2, 4, 5, or 7 months and at other intervening ages are essentially extrapolated values. The test was designed to be compatible at later ages (2 years upwards) with the Stanford–Binet Form L-M and included many Stanford–Binet items (but with more lenient criteria for passing an item). Many other items were similar to the Gesell Scales. The test was designed for children from 2 to 30 months. Five items are presented at each age level, and the test was designed specifically to measure "intelligence." No personal–social items from the Gesell or gross motor items are included in this test. The test may still be used by some individuals because so-called IQ scores below 50 (the floor of the Bayley) can be obtained.

2.2.12. Fagan Test of Infant Intelligence

In reviewing developmental assessment test data, physicians may encounter references to the Fagan Test of Infant Intelligence (FTII).[62,63] The FTII is a relatively new commercially marketed screening device reported to identify infants at risk for later cognitive deficits. The test is administered between 3 and 7 months of age, and it involves infants' differential fixation to novel, versus familiar, pictures. This visual preference is presumed to indicate that the infant can discriminate between pictures as well as remember a picture seen previously. Data on the infant's developing ability to perceive and retain information are collected, and the assumption is that these same processes are involved in later intelligence tests.

A total of 12 novelty problems are presented. Stimuli consist of pairs of abstract black-and-white patterns and faces. The infant views one of the two components of the stimulus pair and then subsequently is simultaneously presented with both stimuli (one familiar, one novel). A preference (longer visual fixation) for the novel stimulus represents better information processing [i.e., when one stimulus elicits significantly more of the infants' total fixation time ($\geq 53\%$)].

This approach is promising; however, more data are necessary. For example, although reported sensitivity and specificity values in regard to function at 3 years are respectable, various samples were combined, and the "gold standard" for measuring 3-year IQ varied. Moreover, of the samples, only 15 out of 128 children were delayed, at least one-third of them significantly so. The FTII may be useful as part of an overall test of developmental screening; however, more refinement is necessary before it is appropriate for widespread clinical use. Therefore, at present, this instrument has more research than clinical applications.

2.2.13. Kent Infant Development Scale

The Kent Infant Development Scale[64] (KIDS) is a caregiver report used in the developmental assessment of normal infants up to 12 months of age and handicapped children having a developmental level of 14 months or less. The KIDS surveys 252 behavioral items grouped into five domains: cognitive, language, motor, self-help, and social. In addition to more traditional, developmental items such as walking, drinking from a cup, or playing with hands, the KIDS includes other unique items such as "gets startled by sudden voices or noises," "shows jealousy," or "remembers where things are kept in the house." Caretakers are provided with three scoring options: (1) yes, can do it, (2) yes, used to do it but outgrew it, or

(3) no, cannot do it yet. A profile sheet is provided in which the Developmental Age (DA) can be plotted for each of the five domains, as well as the Full-Scale Score (see Figure 2.4). This feature is quite helpful in discussing the infant's current levels of development or rate of change. To avoid parental biases, items are not presented in expected developmental sequence. However, the developmental sequence of items is listed in the manual. The KIDS can be hand or computer scored. It was originally designed as a research instrument but is a useful screening instrument for developmental delay.

The KIDS, normed on 450 infants, is psychometrically sound[65] and correlates well with the Bayley Scales ($r = 0.59$–0.72). In regard to diagnostic classification, agreement with the Bayley is greater than 90%.

The major drawback of the KIDS is the fact that data are entirely reliant on informant report; this raises the possibility of bias. Therefore, in light of the limitations of reported versus observed behaviors, the KIDS should not be used as the sole evaluation instrument. Clinicians may elect to use a direct observational procedure in order to score items, particularly in cases where the child can be observed over a sustained period of time (e.g., in daycare settings). The KIDS is particularly useful in working with high-risk or handicapped children.

2.2.14. Miller Assessment for Preschoolers

The stated purpose of the Miller Assessment for Preschoolers[66] (MAP) is to identify preschoolers who are at risk for developmental delay. This well-standardized assessment instrument was normed on 4000 children and is applicable from ages 2.9 to 6 years. The MAP contains 27 items and requires 25 to 35 min for administration. Items are grouped into five performance areas: (1) Neural foundations (ten items), (2) Coordination (seven items), (3) Verbal (four items), (4) Nonverbal (five items), and (5) Complex tasks (four items). Therefore, abilities assessed fall into three main conceptual categories: Sensory and motor, Cognitive, and Combined. A summary, "overall" percentile is computed, as are five Index percentiles.

- *Sensory and motor*. This category includes Foundations and Coordination. Foundations consist of basic motor tasks and awareness of sensations (position, movement, touch). Many of these items are included in a standard neurological examination (e.g., stereogenesis, finger localization, hand–nose, Romberg). The Coordination subtests measure gross motor, fine motor, and oral motor

85

KIDScale Profile Sheet

Name: _____   Date of Birth: _____

Date Test 1: _____   CA (mos.): _____

Date Test 2: _____   CA (mos.): _____

Date Test 3: _____   CA (mos.): _____

DA In Months	Full	Cognitive	Motor	Language	Self-Help	Social
>15.0	249	50	79	38	39	50
14.5	245	49	78	37	38	49
14.0	241	48	77	36	37	48
13.5	236		76	35	36	47
13.0	231	47	74	34	35	46
12.5	226	46	72	33	34	45
12.0	221	45	71	32	33	44
11.5	215	44	69	31	32	43
11.0	209	43	67	29	31	42
10.5	203	42	65	28	30	41
10.0	196	41	62	27	29	40
9.5	189	39	60	26	28	38
9.0	182	38	58	25	27	37
8.5	174	37	55	24	25	35
8.0	167	35	52	23	24	34
7.5	158	33	50	22	23	32
7.0	150	32	47	21	22	31
6.5	141	30	44	19	20	29
6.0	132	28	41	18	19	28
5.5	123	26	37	17	18	25
5.0	113	24	34	16	16	24
4.5	103	22	30	15	15	22
4.0	93	20	27	14	13	20
3.5	82	17	23	12	12	18
3.0	71	15	19	11	10	16
2.5	60	13	15	10	9	13
<2.0	49	10	11	9	7	11

	Full	Cognitive	Motor	Language	Self-Help	Social	Standard
Test 1 Raw Score / DA:							
Test 2 Raw Score / DA:							
Test 3 Raw Score / DA:							

FIGURE 2.4. KIDScale Profile Sheet (1990 norms). From the Kent Infant Development Scale (KIDS). (Copyright 1981 by Kent Developmental Metrics. Reproduced by permission.)

functions (tower building, tongue movements, articulation). Some items combine functions (walking line, rapid alternating movements).

- *Cognitive.* Includes verbal and nonverbal areas. Verbal items evaluate memory, sequencing, comprehension, association, and verbal expression (general information, following directions, sentence and digit repetition). Nonverbal functions assess memory, sequencing, and visual performance (e.g., block tapping, object memory, puzzles).
- *Combined abilities.* This area combines sensory, motor, and cognitive abilities that are required for interpretation of spatial–visual information (block designs, mazes, draw-a-person, imitation of postures).

Six different color-coded record forms are provided. On each form, long rectangular blocks contain intervals that are colored red, yellow, or green. A score falling in the red area indicates that the child is functioning at or below the fifth percentile for his/her age group. Scores in the yellow interval are between the sixth and 25th percentile, whereas those in the green area are above the 25th percentile. Children scoring in the red area need further evaluation, those in the yellow should be monitored carefully, whereas children falling in the green area are within normal limits.

The MAP is an assessment, not a screening test, and does not equally identify children at all levels.[67] More specifically, the test is geared toward identifying children with potential learning problems who are functioning below the 25th percentile; its discriminative abilities in separating out levels of "normal" children are not nearly as precise. In the manual, emphasis is placed on making the test fun for children and allowing the child to feel that he or she is doing well, even if functioning is below normal. The test can be administered by physicians, psychologists, occupational/physical therapists, and other allied professionals. In clinical practice, the test is very useful in identifying mild and moderate "preacademic" problems, and it has been recommended by some as being much more accurate than the DDST in that regard.[67]

2.2.15. FirstSTEP: Screening Test for Evaluating Preschoolers

The FirstSTEP[68] is a screener for the Miller Assessment for Preschoolers and takes approximately 15 min to administer. The short amount of time required for administration makes the FirstSTEP attractive for office practice. The FirstSTEP consists of 12 subtests, arranged in five domains (see discussion of MAP 2.1.14). However, the composite score is comprised of information obtained in only three areas: Cognition, Communication, and Motor. Based on test results, children are classified as: (1) falling within normal limits, (2) questionable (mild to moderate developmental delays), or (3) at risk (significant developmental delays). Scoring sheets are arranged in three levels: (1) 2.9 to 3.8 years, (2) 3.9 to 4.8 years, and (3), 4.9 to 6.2 years. There also are an optional Socio–Emotional Scale (examiner-observed behavior checklist), a Parent/Teacher Rating Checklist, and an Adaptive Behavior Checklist. The Socio–Emotional and Parent/ Teacher Checklists survey attention/activity levels, social interactions, personal traits, and serious behavior problems. The Adaptive Behavior Checklist surveys activities of daily living, self-control, relationships and interactions, and functioning in the community. (These optional checklists are not included in the final score.)

The FirstSTEP has just become available; as a result, there is little clinical information available at this time. Nonetheless, it appears to be promising in regard to application in office practice.

2.3. SUMMARY

As was mentioned in the beginning of this chapter, this list of developmental screening and assessment instruments is not exhaustive. For example, the Alpern–Boll Developmental Profile II,[69] the Brigance Early Preschool Screen,[70] or the Mullen Scales of Early Learning,[71] also used in clinical practice, are not discussed here in detail. The reader is advised that exclusion of these and other tests does not necessarily reflect negatively on these instruments.

Selection of an evaluation instrument will depend on the reasons for testing and the type(s) of information desired. Practitioners may want to screen large groups of children or instead might prefer to concentrate on testing only those patients who appear developmentally at risk. Moreover, clinicians must appreciate the fact that all tests do not measure the same functional areas; therefore, screening and assessment instruments must be chosen carefully, depending on the specific questions to be answered. Consideration of areas of function outlined in the next two chapters (language and adaptive) also is necessary.

REFERENCES

1. Smith, R. D., 1978, The use of developmental screening tests by primary care physicians, *J. Pediatr.* **93:**524–527.

2. Carr, J., and Stephen, E., 1964, Pediatricians and developmental tests, *Dev. Med. Child. Neurol.* **6:**614.
3. Dobos, A. D., Dworkin, P. H., and Bernstein, B., 1992, Pediatricians; approaches to developmental problems: 15 years later, *Am. J Dis. Child.* **146:**484.
4. Meisels, S. J., and Provence, S., 1989, *Screening and Assessment: Guidelines for Identifying Young Disabled and Developmentally Vulnerable Children and Their Families*, National Center for Clinical Infant Programs, Washington, DC.
5. Aylward, G. P., 1992, The relationship between environmental risk and developmental outcome, *J. Dev. Behav. Pediatr.* **13:**222–229.
6. Dworkin, P. H., 1989, Developmental screening—expecting the impossible? *Pediatrics* **83:**619–622.
7. Whitmore, K., and Bax, M., 1988, Screening or examining? *Dev. Med. Child. Neurol.* **30:** 673–676.
8. Dworkin, P. H., 1992, Developmental screening: (Still) expecting the impossible? *Pediatrics* **89:**1253–1255.
9. Illingworth, R. S., 1990, *Basic Developmental Screening 0–4 Years*, ed. 5, Blackwell Scientific Publications, London.
10. McCue-Horwitz, S., Leaf, P. J., Leventhal, J. M., et al., 1992, Identification and management of psychosocial and developmental problems in community-based, primary care pediatric practices, *Pediatrics* **89:**480–485.
11. Rosenbaum, M. S., Chua-Lim, C., Wilhite, J., and Mankad, V. P., 1983, Applicability of the Denver Prescreening Developmental Questionnaire in a low-income population, *Pediatrics* **71:**359–363.
12. Palfrey, J. S., Singer, J. D., Walker, D. K., and Butler, J. A., 1987, Early identification of children's special needs: A study in five metropolitan communities, *J. Pediatr.* **111:** 651–659.
13. Bagnato, S. J., 1992, Assessment for early intervention: Best practices with young children and families, *Child Asses. News* **2:**1–10.
14. Frankenburg, W. K., and Dodds, J. B., 1967, The Denver Developmental Screening Test, *J. Pediatr.* **71:**181–191.
15. Frankenburg, W. K., Goldstein, A. D., and Camp, B. W., 1971, The revised Denver Developmental Screening Test: Its accuracy as a screening instrument, *J. Pediatr.* **79:** 988–995.
16. Frankenburg, W. K., Fandal, A. W., Sciarillo, W., and Burgess, D., 1981, The newly abbreviated and revised Denver Developmental Screening Test, *J. Pediatr.* **99:**995–999.
17. Frankenburg, W. K., Ker, C. Y., Engelke, S., Schaefer, E. S., and Thornton, S. M., 1988, Validation of key Denver Developmental Screening test items: A preliminary study, *J. Pediatr.* **112:**560–566.
18. Meisels, S. J., 1989, Can developmental screening tests identify children who are developmentally at risk? *Pediatrics* **83:**578–585.
19. Frankenburg, W. K., Chen, J., and Thornton, S. M., 1988, Common pitfalls in the evaluation of developmental screening tests, *J. Pediatr.* **113:**1110–1113.
20. Cadman, D., Chambers, L. W., Walter, S. D., Feldman, W., et al., 1984, The usefulness of the Denver Developmental test to predict kindergarten problems in a general community population, *Am. J. Public Health* **74:**1093–1097.
21. Sturner, R. A., Green, J. A., and Funk, S. G., 1985, Preschool Denver Developmental Screening Test as a predictor of later school problems, *J. Pediatr.* **107:**615–621.
22. Frankenburg, W. K., Dodds, J. B., and Fandal, A. W., 1973, *Denver Developmental Screening Test Manual/Workbook for Nursing and Paramedical Personnel*, LADOCA Publishing, Denver.

23. Frankenburg, W. K., Dodds, J., Archer, P., Bresnick, B., and Shapiro, H., 1990, The Denver II: Revision and restandardization of the DDST, *Am. J. Dis. Child.* **144**:446.
24. Frankenburg, W. K., Dodds, J., Archer, P., Bresnick, B., et al., 1990, *Denver II Screening Manual*, Denver Developmental Materials, Denver.
25. Frankenburg, W. K., Dodds, J., Archer, P., et al., 1992, The Denver II: A major revision and restandardization of the Denver Developmental Screening Test, *Pediatrics* **89**: 91–97.
26. Glascoe, F. P., Byrne, K. E., Ashford, L. G., et al., 1992, Accuracy of the Denver-II in developmental screening, *Pediatrics* **89**:1221–1225.
27. Frankenburg, W. K., van Doorninck, W. J., Liddell, T. N., and Dick, N. P., 1976, The Denver Prescreening Developmental Questionnaire (PDQ), *Pediatrics* **57**:744–753.
28. Frankenburg, W. K., Fandal, A. W., and Thornton, S. M., 1987, Revision of Denver Prescreening Developmental Questionnaire, *J. Pediatr.* **110**:653–657.
29. Bayley, N., 1969, *Bayley Scales of Infant Development*. Psychological Corporation, New York.
30. Cattell, P., 1960, *The Measurement of Intelligence in Infants and Young Children*, Psychological Corporation, New York.
31. Aylward, G. P., Gustafson, N., Verhulst, S. J., and Colliver, J., 1987, Consistency in the diagnosis of cognitive, motor and neurologic function over the first three years, *J. Pediatr. Psychol.* **12**:77–98.
32. Aylward, G. P., 1987, Developmental assessment: Caveats and a cry for quality control, *J. Pediatr.* **110**:253–254.
33. Bayley, N., 1993, *The Bayley II Manual*, The Psychological Corporation, San Antonio, TX.
34. Gesell, A., and Amatruda, C., 1941, *Developmental Diagnosis*. Paul B. Hoeber, New York.
35. Knobloch, H., Stevens, F., and Malone, A. F., 1980, *Manual of Developmental Diagnosis*, Harper & Row, New York.
36. McCall, R. B., 1982, A hard look at stimulating and predicting development: The cases of bonding and screening, *Pediatr. Rev.* **3**:205–212.
37. Aylward, G. P., 1992, *Bayley Infant Neurodevelopmental Screen. Standardization Manual*, The Psychological Corporation, San Antonio.
38. Aylward, G. P., 1994, Update on early developmental neuropsychologic assessment: The Early Neuropsychologic Optimality Rating Scales, in: *Advances in Child Neuropsychology*, Volume 2 (M. G. Tramontana and S. R. Hooper, eds.), Springer-Verlag, New York, pp. 172–200.
39. Aylward, G. P., Verhulst, S. J., and Bell, S., 1988, The Early Neuropsychologic Optimality Rating Scale (ENORS-9): A new developmental follow-up technique, *J. Dev. Behav. Pediatr.* **9**:140–146.
40. Aylward, G. P., Verhulst, S. J., and Bell, S., 1988, The 18-month Early Neuropsychologic Optimality Rating Scale (ENORS-18): A predictive assessment instrument, *Dev. Neuropsychol.* **4**:47–61.
41. Aylward, G. P., Verhulst, S. J., and Bell, S., 1992, Bayley Infant Neurodevelopmental Screener (BINS) prediction profiles in outcome of at-risk infants, *Am. J. Dis. Child.* **146**:464.
42. Aylward, G. P., Verhulst, S. J., and Bell, S., 1992, Prediction of outcome in at-risk infants: Application of the Bayley Infant Neurodevelopmental Screen to the Risk Route Model, *Dev. Med. Child. Neurol.* **34**(66):33.
43. Prechtl, A. F. R., 1980, The optimality concept, *Early Hum. Dev.* **4**:201–205.
44. Milani-Comparetti, A., and Gidoni, E. A., 1967, Pattern analyses of motor development and its disorders, *Dev. Med. Child. Neurol.* **9**:625–630.
45. Milani-Comparetti, A., and Gidoni, E. A., 1967, Routine developmental examination in normal and retarded children, *Dev. Med. Child. Neurol.* **9**:631–636.

46. Ellison, P. H., Browning, C. A., Larson, B., and Denny, J., 1983, Development of a scoring system for the Milani–Comparetti and Gidoni method of assessing neurologic abnormality in infancy, *Phys. Ther.* **63:**1414–1423.
47. Stuberg, W. A., Dehne, P. R., Miedaner, J. A., et al., 1987, *Milani–Comparetti Motor Development Screening Test: Test Manual*, C. Louis Meyer Children's Rehabilitation Institute, University of Nebraska Medical Center, Omaha.
48. Stuberg, W. A., White, P. J., Miedaner, J. A., and Dehne, P. R., 1989, Item reliability of the Milani–Comparetti Motor Development Screening Test, *Phys. Ther.* **69:**328–335.
49. Newborg, J., Stock, J. R., Wnek, L., Guidubaldi, J., and Svinicki, J., 1984, *The Battelle Developmental Inventory*, DLM Teaching Resources, Allen, TX.
50. Harrington, R., 1985, Battelle Developmental Inventory, in: *Test Critiques*, Volume II (D. J. Keyser and R. C. Sweetland, eds.), Test Corporation of America, Kansas City, MO, pp. 72–82.
51. Sexton, D., McLean, M., Boyd, R. D., Thompson, B., and McCormick, K., 1988, Criterion-related validity of a new standardized developmental measure for use with infants who are handicapped, *Meas. Eval. Couns. Dev.* **21:**16–24.
52. Burnett, D. W., 1992, Review of the Battelle Developmental Inventory Screening Test, in: *11th Mental Measurements Yearbook* (J. J. Kramer and J. Close-Conoley, eds.), University of Nebraska Press, Lincoln, pp. 65–67.
53. Boyd, R. D., 1989, What a difference a day makes: Age-related discontinuities and the Battelle Developmental Inventory, *J. Early Intervent.* **13:**114–119.
54. Ershler, J., and Elliott, S. N., 1992, Review of the Battelle Developmental Inventory Screening Test, in: *11th Mental Measurements Yearbook* (J. J. Kramer and J. Close-Conoley, eds.), University of Nebraska Press, Lincoln, pp. 67–72.
55. Elliott, C. D., 1990, *Differential Ability Scales. Introductory and Technical Handbook*, The Psychological Corporation, New York.
56. Aylward, G. P., 1992, Review of the Differential Ability Scales, in: *11th Mental Measurements Yearbook* (J. J. Kramer and J. Close-Conoley, eds.), University of Nebraska Press, Lincoln, pp. 281–282.
57. Elliott, C. D., Daniel, M. H., and Guiton, G. W., 1991, Preschool cognitive assessment with the Differential Ability Scales, in: *The Psychoeducational Assessment of Preschool Children*, ed. 2 (B. A. Bracken, ed.), Allyn and Bacon, Boston, pp. 133–153.
58. McCarthy, D., 1972, *McCarthy Scales of Children's Abilities*, The Psychological Corporation, New York.
59. Bracken, B. A., 1991, The assessment of preschool children with the McCarthy Scales of Children's Abilities, in: *The Psychoeducational Assessment of Preschool Children*, ed. 2 (B. A. Bracken, ed.), Allyn and Bacon, Boston, pp. 53–85.
60. Valencia, R. R., 1990, Clinical assessment of young children with the McCarthy Scales of Children's Abilities, in: *Handbook of Psychological and Educational Assessment of Children* (C. C. Reynolds and R. W. Kamphaus, eds.), Guilford Press, New York, pp. 209–258.
61. Kaufman, A. S., 1977, A McCarthy short form for rapid screening of preschool, kindergarten, and first-grade children, *Contemp. Ed. Psychol.* **2:**149–157.
62. Fagan, J. F., Singer, L. T., Montie, J. E., and Shepherd, P. A., 1986, Selective screening device for the early detection of normal or delayed cognitive development in infants at risk for later mental retardation, *Pediatrics* **78:**1021–1026.
63. Fagan, J. F., and Montie, J. E., 1988, The behavioral assessment of cognitive well-being in the infant, in: *Understanding Mental Retardation: Research Accomplishments and New Frontiers* (J. Kavanaugh, ed.), Paul H. Brooks, Baltimore, pp. 207–221.
64. Reuter, J., and Bickett, L., 1985, *Kent Infant Development Scale (KIDS)*, ed. 2, Kent Developmental Metrics, Kent, OH.

65. Feiring, C., 1989, Review of the Kent Infant Development Scale second edition, in: *The Tenth Mental Measurements Yearbook* (J. Close-Conoley and J. Kramer, eds.), University of Nebraska Press, Lincoln, pp. 415–418.

66. Miller, L. J., 1988, *Miller Assessment for Preschoolers*, The Psychological Corporation, San Antonio.

67. DeLoria, D. J., 1985, Review of the Miller Assessment for Preschoolers, in: *The Ninth Mental Measurements Yearbook* (J. V. Mitchell, ed.), University of Nebraska Press, Lincoln, pp. 56–57.

68. Miller, L. J., 1993, *FirstSTEP: Screening Test for Evaluating Preschoolers*, The Psychological Corporation, San Antonio.

69. Alpern, G. D., Boll, T. J., and Shearer, M. S., 1984, *Developmental Profile II*, Western Psychological Services, Los Angeles.

70. Brigance, A. H., 1990, *Brigance Early Preschool Screen for Two-Year-Old and Two-and-a-Half-Year-Old Children*, Curriculum Associates, North Billerica, MA.

71. Mullen, E. M., 1985, *Manual for the Infant Mullen Scales of Early Learning*. T.O.T.A.L. Child, Cranston, RI.

3 ❋ Evaluation of Language Function

3.1. INTRODUCTION

Language function must be assessed in the evaluation of any child with suspected developmental delay. Language probably is the single most important cognitive achievement before 5 years of age, and it provides the foundation for later accomplishments. Language delays are often the first indication or marker of underlying cognitive impairment; assessment techniques useful to the primary-care physician are listed in Table 3.1. The majority of these assessment instruments can be administered in the physician's office. It should be emphasized that many of the developmental assessment techniques cited in Chapter 2 also include language components.

Early and reliable identification of children with language impairments is important not only to provide early intervention but also because these children are at significant risk for subsequent educational, social, emotional, and behavioral problems.[1] As a result, there is increasing awareness of the seriousness of delayed language in young children. Indeed, in a study of children who manifested early language impairments (onset before 5 years of age), only 5% were functioning at a grade-appropriate reading level at age 9; moreover, two-thirds were receiving some type of learning-disabilities assistance.[2] It has been shown that in later childhood and older, from 28% to 75% of children whose preschool language was impaired continue to exhibit residual language/speech problems, and 52% to 95% show impairment in reading achievement.[3,4] There also is recent evidence that between the ages of 3 to 5 years there is an "illusory" recovery in children with early language delay. This apparently "normal" function again reverts back to delay by the end of the second grade.[5] It has been suggested that this change may reflect testing artifacts.

Speech and language are both components of communication.[6]

TABLE 3.1. Listing of Language Assessment Instruments

Language assessment	Language area assessed			Type		Appropriate for office use	
	Expressive	Receptive	Articulation	Screen	Detailed	Yes	No
Peabody Picture Vocabulary Test-Revised (PPVT-R)		X			X	X	
Early Language Milestone Scale (ELMS)	X	X	X	X		X	
Preschool Language Scale (PLS)/Preschool Language Scale-3	X	X	X		X		X
Boehm Test of Basic Concepts-Revised/ Preschool Version		X			X		X
Receptive–Expressive Emergent Language Scale (REEL)	X	X		X		X	
Arizona Articulation Proficiency Scale-Revised			X	X			X
Northwestern Syntax Screening Test	X	X		X			X
Clinical Linguistic and Auditory Milestone Scale (CLAMS)	X	X		X		X	

Speech is the overt, motor behavior that is dependent on physiological and neuromuscular development; language is knowledge of a code or system of rules in which ideas, events, or objects are represented by means of signals or symbols.[6] It is possible for a child to have impaired speech but intact language, and vice versa.

The most recent findings in the area of "developmental neurolinguistics"[7] suggest that there are several *sensitive periods* for language development. Languages learned between birth and approximately 7 years of age are likely to be expressed with a native-sounding accent (this is also the period where the bulk of language is mastered).[7] There is a second, "sensitive" interval that extends through adolescence, after which the ability to learn language declines significantly.

In terms of laterality, neither left- nor right-hemisphere lesions incurred during infancy produce lasting effects on language development. Obviously, there is central nervous system plasticity, which allows for cerebral reorganization. However, mechanisms in the left hemisphere are activated by speech as early as 3 months of age, with the left planum being larger than the right by the third trimester of fetal life. "Vocal prosody" (variations of vocal pitch, tempo, loudness) and "vocal affect" (expression of mood, emotion, and attitude) are interpreted in the right hemisphere.[7] "Linguistic prosody" (stressing different syllables of the same word in order to differentiate noun and verb forms or adjective–noun combinations) and identification of spoken and written words are monitored by the left hemisphere. Therefore, problems in understanding or expressing language may emanate from damage to *either* hemisphere, depending on the *type* of problem.

In processing information, the stimulus first has to be received (input); it then must be retained (short-term memory), integrated (central processing), and acted upon (output). Language disorders can affect any or all of these functions, and physicians should be sensitive to a child's difficulties in receptive language, central processing, or expressive language. In performing a language assessment, it is critical to recognize that environmental deprivation also can have a major negative impact on language function.[8]

Receptive language disorders include dysfunction in auditory discrimination, auditory blending, auditory sequencing, or auditory memory. Auditory discrimination and/or auditory blending problems may be manifested as a child saying the word "animal" as "aminal," "enemy" as "emeny," or "magazine" as "mazagine." Children with auditory sequencing deficits, when presented with a series of digits or words to recall, may confuse the sequence (e.g., 1, 3, 5, 7 may be repeated as 1, 5, 3, 7). The child with an auditory memory problem might not be able to recall a series of numbers, words, and/or sounds. Central processing disorders are suggested when a child cannot comprehend what is verbalized or derive conceptual meaning from verbal information. Inability to recall the salient aspects of stories told by the examiner to the child may be another indication of a central processing disorder.

Expressive disorders include dysarthria, dyspraxia, and dysnomia. Dysarthria, or difficulty in producing speech because of oral motor problems, essentially reflects poor sound production. Dyspraxia is the difficulty in organizing and producing spoken language despite intact oral motor skills. Although there is no muscle paralysis, and the child can produce appropriate sounds, output is poorly organized. Dysarthria and dyspraxia often occur concurrently. Dysnomia, a problem finding or retrieving words, is associated with the child producing circumlocutions. These word retrieval difficulties often are reflected in a child calling a tree a flower or being able to describe the characteristics of a cat but not being able to name the animal.

Mildly developmentally delayed children typically progress through the same sequence of language development as their normal peers, but at a slower rate. In addition, children with developmental delays show a higher percentage of language disorders. As indicated previously, the receptive language disorders cited often are associated with subsequent learning disabilities. There is approximately a 2:1 male to female ratio in regard to language disorders, and in general speech and language development in males is slower. Practitioners should be cognizant that in a hypothetical sample of 200 children, eight have articulation disorders, two some type of language disorder, one or two stutter, and one has a voice disorder.[9] In regard to causes of speech and/or language delays in children younger than 3 years, developmental delay accounts for approximately 50% of the cases, partial hearing loss 33%, cerebral palsy about 5%, anatomic etiologies less than 2%, oral motor apraxia 5%, and 3% to 4% is attributable to communicative disorders.[9]

Unfortunately, poor psychometric quality exists in many well-known language tests, and age-equivalent scores are misused as measures of language ability.[10] In actuality, standard scores should be utilized (see Chapter 1). Correlations between language tests and other assessment instruments, such as those measuring intelligence, range from $r = 0.50$ to 0.60; however, these correlations may be lower in language-disordered groups.[1] Z scores (see Chapter 1) are rarely reported; therefore, direct comparison between different tests is precluded.[1]

Test batteries, versus single language tests, must be used to differentiate reliably between transient and persistent language impairments. Moreover, because most language tests are not designed for use with handicapped populations, problems with interpretation arise. It is important to distinguish between children with specific language delays and those whose language difficulties are attributable to more pervasive problems in learning or cognitive impairment.[11] Not only is this differentiation necessary for intervention purposes, but prognosis also differs (with the latter group having poorer outcome).[12,13]

A description of selected language assessment techniques follows.

3.2. PEABODY PICTURE VOCABULARY TEST-REVISED

The Peabody Picture Vocabulary Test-Revised[14] (PPVT-R) was developed in 1965 and revised in 1981. This test is versatile, nonthreatening, and useful in the evaluation of language and communication disorders. It was normed on a sample of 4200 subjects and is applicable from ages $2\frac{1}{2}$ years through adulthood. Receptive vocabulary is assessed over 10 to 20 min, during which the child is presented with a series of pictures that portray increasingly difficult words. Each of the 175 PPVT-R plates contains four pictures from which the child is required to select one picture that corresponds to a word named by the examiner. The basal age is eight consecutive correct responses, and the ceiling is six failed out of the last eight. Two interchangeable forms, L and M, are provided, which allows a different vocabulary word to be presented for each page, thereby establishing a retesting format. An example is shown in Figure 3.1.

The mean PPVT-R score is 100 (SD = 15), and scores range from 40 to 160. The 1981 revision provides standard scores, not a deviation IQ, as designated in the earlier version. Percentiles and age equivalents also are provided. The physician should consider 95% confidence limits to range ±14.

The PPVT-R is an excellent test to establish rapport; however, normal children tend to score lower on this task than on the Stanford–Binet or Wechsler scales.[15] Moreover, children from depressed socioeconomic backgrounds or minorities would score lower on the Peabody than on tests such as the Stanford–Binet because of a relative paucity of language stimulation. Children with attention-deficit disorders (ADD) also score lower than their non-ADD counterparts, in part because of impulsivity. The PPVT-R is useful in evaluation of children with speech disorders or physical handicaps such as cerebral palsy, as it measures receptive skills. However, although the PPVT-R yields an estimate of verbal intelligence, it

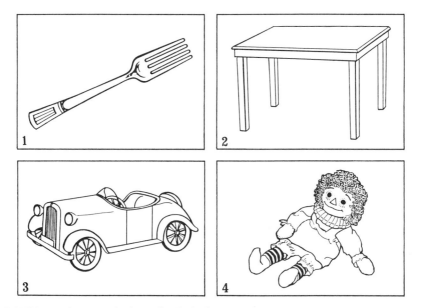

FIGURE 3.1. An example from the Peabody Picture Vocabulary Test-Revised (PPVT-R). (Copyright 1981 American Guidance Service, Inc., 4201 Woodland Road, Circle Pines, MN 55014-1796. All rights reserved.)

is not interchangeable with an IQ test; correlations between the PPVT-R and other measures of intelligence generally are below $r = 0.80$ (a level that is recommended when one measure is used in place of another). An age-appropriate score can help to rule out mental retardation; however, a low score by itself should not be used to make the diagnosis of developmental delay.

3.3. EARLY LANGUAGE MILESTONE SCALE

The Early Language Milestone Scale[16] (ELMS) is valuable in the "evaluation of speech and language development during infancy and early childhood" (p. 5). The ELMS usually is utilized for children aged 0 to 36 months. However, it can also be used in older, developmentally delayed children whose level of language function is below 36 months.

Items in the ELMS are grouped into three areas: auditory expressive, auditory receptive, and visual. The auditory expressive area assesses early language and speech behaviors and includes single words, phrases, and sentences. In addition, prelinguistic behaviors such as cooing, reciprocal vocalization, and babbling are measured. The auditory receptive realm (which assesses responses to sounds and comprehension of simple commands) involves execution of commands, recognition of sounds, and localization of auditory stimuli in space. The visual area assesses responses to visual stimuli and some gesture behaviors; it includes prelinguistic behaviors such as visual fixation, visual tracking, visual recognition of parents, and gestures. Conceptually, the culmination of visual language development is considered to be reflected in the child using his index finger to point to desired objects.

The ELMS consists of 41 items and is formatted in a manner similar to the DDST (see Figure 3.2). Items can be passed by history (H), direct testing (T), or incidental observation (O); most are scored by history or observation. An age line is drawn, and items that are passed by 50% or more of children of the same age are administered; the basal is three passes. A drinking cup, spoon, crayon, rubber ball, and wooden cube are required for administration of the test. All three areas (expressive, receptive, and visual) must be passed in order for a child to be considered to have normal language development.

The ELMS was normed on 191 children, 96 males and 95 females; 80% of the subjects were Caucasian. This suggests that the number of children used at each age was rather small. Moreover, most were English-speaking, and the majority were from middle-class backgrounds. When applied to a sample of 119 children who were at high risk for the presence of develop-

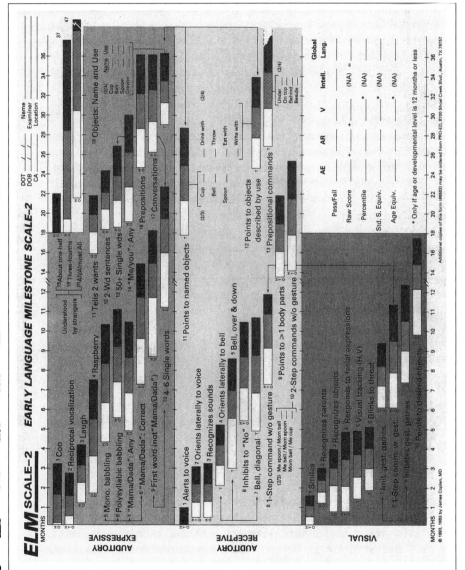
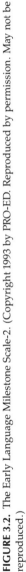

FIGURE 3.2. The Early Language Milestone Scale-2. (Copyright 1993 by PRO-ED. Reproduced by permission. May not be reproduced.)

mental disabilities, the ELMS was 97% sensitive and 93% specific in detecting language delay.[17]

The test is a helpful screening tool for use by the practitioner, particularly because of the relative weakness of the language component of the DDST.[18] Some concern has been expressed by clinicians familiar with the ELMS that sensitivity may be low. Correlations between the ELMS and the PPVT-R[14] (both administered at 30 months of age) are approximately $r = 0.51$, suggesting moderate concurrent validity. Sensitivity, using the Bayley Scales (BSID) as the "gold standard," ranges from 50% to 63%; specificity values range from 71% to 100%. False negatives are more frequent in the 0- to 12-month age range; therefore, the ELMS is recommended for the children in the 25- to 36-month age interval.[19,20] In general, there is a 38% to 50% rate of false negatives (underreferrals) with this instrument, and the validity of results increases with multiple administrations. This suggests the need for rescreening with the ELMS on a periodic basis.[19,20] Recently a point-scoring technique for the ELMS has been developed, making it possible to express the child's score on the ELM Scale as a percentile value for chronological age.[21] This technique has been incorporated into the second edition (ELM Scale-2). The ELM Scale has been incorporated into the *Guidelines for Hearing and Language Screening of Young Children in Physicians' Offices.*[22]

A helpful gross screening item for the practitioner, included in the ELMS, is the suggestion that children should be 50% intelligible by 2 years of age, 75% intelligible by age 3, and 100% intelligible by age 4. Intelligibility is assessed simply by asking the parent how much of their child's speech can be understood by a stranger: less than half, one-half, three-fourths, or almost all.[23]

3.4. PRESCHOOL LANGUAGE SCALE/PRESCHOOL LANGUAGE SCALE-3

The individually administered Preschool Language Scale/Preschool Language Scale-3[24,25] (PLS/PLS-3) can be used for children ages 1 to 6 years, although it is most appropriately administered between the ages of $1\frac{1}{2}$ and $4\frac{1}{2}$ years. The test measures auditory comprehension (receptive verbal skills) and verbal ability (expressive skills). Each area is tested separately, and discrepancies between auditory comprehension and verbal ability are important diagnostically. An auditory comprehension age, verbal ability age, and a language age are obtained. The language age is simply the average of the verbal ability and auditory comprehension age equivalents.

Test materials include the PLS picture book, 12 1-inch colored blocks, a piece of coarse sandpaper, six coins, and a watch.

The PLS contains four auditory and four verbal items at $\frac{1}{2}$-year intervals up to 5 years and yearly thereafter. Areas evaluated include sensory discrimination, logical thinking, grammar and vocabulary, memory and attention span, temporal/spatial relations, and self-image. Auditory comprehension items include knowledge of body parts, following directions, comparing size, prepositions, and colors. Verbal ability items involve tasks such as naming animals, pronouncing sounds, repeating digits, and conversing. An articulation component is also incorporated in the test.

The PLS is very helpful in isolating specific areas of language dysfunction, particularly in the early childhood age range. Specific emphasis should be placed on discrepancies between the receptive- and expressive-language age equivalents.

The PLS-3[25] contains an optional articulation screener and allows the examiner to give credit for an item if the behavior was observed in spontaneous interactions. The PLS-3 can be used with older children with developmental delays, and it meets PL 99-457 (IDEA) guidelines for determining eligibility for programs such as Head Start. A Spanish version is also available. The PLS-3 correlates moderately with the BSID-II MDI ($r = 0.52$); correlations with the PDI are lower ($r = 0.29$–0.38).

3.5. BOEHM TEST OF BASIC CONCEPTS-REVISED/BOEHM TEST OF BASIC CONCEPTS-PRESCHOOL VERSION

The Boehm Test of Basic Concepts/Boehm Test-Revised[26,27] (BTBC-R), which consists of 50 basic concepts, can be administered individually or in a group format. The BTBC-R is primarily helpful for assessing children in the kindergarten through elementary setting (grade 2). The Preschool Version[27] consists of 52 items, applicable to children ages 3-0 to 5-0 years. The Boehm test is particularly useful in identifying children who are deficient in the ability to understand basic concepts that may be used in the "directions" portions of curriculum materials.

There are two booklets, each requiring approximately 15 min to administer. Concepts such as space (location, direction, dimensions), quantity (and number), time (after, never), and miscellaneous concepts (different, other) are assessed. Essentially, the child's ability to understand language concepts is measured, as are the abilities to comprehend and follow simple instructions. The child is requested to mark the correct answer from visual displays in response to inquiries from the examiner about concepts such as "away from," "next to," "inside," "some but not many," "most," "between," "nearest," and "equal." For example, the child is presented with a grouping of three pictures: (1) a dog next to a box, (2) a dog lying down, and (3) a dog sitting on top of a box. The child is then asked to mark the picture depicting "the dog is on the box." The test is sensitive to receptive language dysfunction. A Spanish version is also available.

The Boehm Test of Basic Concepts—Preschool Version[27] (BTBC-PV), normed on 433 children, is a downward extension of the BTBC-R. The test is designed to identify language difficulties in preschool screenings. Only three items overlap with the BTBC-R, and age norms are used on this test (only grade norms are used on the BTBC-R). The Preschool Version also evaluates relational concepts involving characteristics of persons and objects. These concepts include: size (e.g., tallest), direction (e.g., up), position in space (under), quantity (many), and time (e.g., after). There are five warm-up items, and each of the 26 concepts is presented twice, producing a total of 52 items. The child is shown a picture and is requested to respond to a question about the picture by pointing to the correct response. A score of "2," "1," or "0" is then assigned for each concept. A score of 2 means that the child is familiar with the concept and its meaning, whereas a 1 or 0 indicates the need for further instruction on the concept. T-scores and percentiles (see Chapter 1) are provided, but age equivalents are not.

The BTBC-PV is related significantly to the Peabody Picture Vocabulary Test ($r = 0.57–0.63$); however, there is little research to date regarding prediction of later academic achievement. Nonetheless, it is useful in clinical practice.

3.6. RECEPTIVE–EXPRESSIVE EMERGENT LANGUAGE SCALE

The Receptive–Expressive Emergent Language Scale[28] (REEL Scale) is a language-screening test that is applicable from birth to 36 months. The 132-item scale is basically a checklist of receptive and expressive language skills that develop over the first 3 years. It is based on a report by a parent or individual who has daily contact with the child, and takes approximately 15 min to administer. Items are grouped in blocks of six (three receptive and three expressive) at 1-month intervals over the first year, 2-month intervals over the second year, and 3-month periods between 2 and 3 years. The child is considered to pass an age level if he/she passes two out of three receptive or two out of three expressive items in that respective block. Reciprocally, the ceiling is failure of two out of three items at a given age. Three scores are derived: receptive and expressive language quotients and an overall language quotient. In addition, receptive, expressive, and combined expressive and receptive language ages are obtained.

Receptive language items include following simple commands (10–11 months), production of verbal responses upon request (11–12 months), recognition of body parts (14–16 months), carrying out two instructions in a row (16–18 months), and recognition of new words each day (20–22 months). Sample expressive items include use of gestures (8–9 months), jargon (9–10 months), consistent use of five or more words (12–14 months), word combinations (20–22), and reference to self by the child using his/her own name (22–24 months).

The REEL Scale was normed on a longitudinal sample of 50 children from environments that provided enhanced language stimulation. Therefore, children from depressed socioeconomic environments are probably at a distinct disadvantage for scoring well on the REEL. Moreover, there is concern that the results of this test are heavily dependent upon the interviewing skills of the test administrator. The questions posed to the caretaker should be open-ended versus simply requiring a yes or no answer. The accuracy of parental report is often subject to question, and this detracts from the utility of this test instrument. The REEL Scale appears most useful for screening during the first 12 to 18 months, whereas other evaluation techniques are more desirable at older ages.

3.7. ARIZONA ARTICULATION PROFICIENCY SCALE-REVISED/ ARIZONA ARTICULATION PROFICIENCY SCALE- SECOND EDITION

The Arizona Articulation Proficiency Scale-Revised[29,30] (AAPS), normed on more than 5000 individuals, is administered to children in the 1.5- to 13-year age range, but it is particularly useful in early childhood assessment. The AAPS requires 10 to 15 min to administer and consists of 48 picture test cards and a 25-item sentence test. This articulation test was designed to detect misarticulations and thereby identify children who are in need of speech therapy.

The child is required to name pictures (black-and-white line drawings) shown by the examiner, who records whether the child can produce chronologically age-appropriate initial and ending consonant sounds and vowels and diphthongs contained within words. Sounds are gauged in regard to "difficulty" (in terms of the sequence of their developmental mastery); e.g., "m," "b," and "p" sounds are much easier to master than are "s," "l," "r," and "th" sounds. Age of phoneme mastery on the AAPS was defined as the earliest age at which 90% of the particular age group achieved mastery of the phoneme. Sounds are therefore assigned values ranging from 0.5 (e.g., *t*ree, *p*ig, *c*up), to 3.5 (trai*n*, fu*n*) or 4.0 (ca*t*, ha*t*). The consonant and vowel values are then summed and subtracted from 100. The author provides a rating scale of normal, moderate, or severe articulation problems for these scores, based on age norms (in $\frac{1}{2}$-year increments from $1\frac{1}{2}$ to 6 years and yearly from 6 through 12).

The AAPS instrument probably can be administered in an office setting and is valuable in the detection of speech problems. However, the developers suggest that the test is geared toward communication-disorders specialists.

3.8. NORTHWESTERN SYNTAX SCREENING TEST

The Northwestern Syntax Screening Text[31] provides a measure of receptive and expressive syntactic competence in children aged 3 years to approximately 8 years. Understanding of prepositions, pronouns, plurals, negatives, verb tenses, possessives, and questions ("who–what–where," yes/no) can be assessed in approximately 10 to 15 min.

In the receptive section, 20 pairs of sentences are presented, and the child is required to select the appropriate picture (out of four) that corresponds to the sentence. For example, "the boy is sitting" and "the boy is not sitting" would be presented, with the child having to respond accordingly.

In the expressive section, two sentences are presented that describe each of two pictures on a page (20 pairs), e.g., "the baby is sleeping" or "the baby is not sleeping." The child is asked to repeat each sentence. This section of the screening instrument is particularly helpful in cases where the child may be able to repeat sentences but be unable to comprehend the message within the sentence. This discrepancy would be highly useful in the diagnostic formulation.

The physician should keep in mind that scores on this test may be affected by environmental factors such as being reared in a depressed socioeconomic household. The instrument only measures syntax and therefore does not measure speech sounds or vocabulary. A child with severe language delay or mental retardation may score low on both the receptive and expressive sections. However, the child who can adequately repeat what he/she hears, in an echolalic fashion, may perform well expressively but do poorly on the receptive section. This test is best administered by a specialist skilled in speech/language assessments.

3.9. CLINICAL LINGUISTIC AND AUDITORY MILESTONE SCALE

The Clinical Linguistic and Auditory Milestone Scale[32] (CLAMS) is a 41-item language screening test, primarily scored by use of parental report (only seven items are elicited). The screening test, which takes 5 min or less to administer, was standardized on 381 normal children. Items were selected because they reflected milestones in language acquisition.

Test items are grouped monthly from 1 to 12 months, in 3-month intervals from 12 to 24 months, and in 6-month blocks from 24 to 36 months. A total of 18 age groupings is provided. The number of items at each age varies from one to six. Sample items include: orients to voice, uses "dada" nonspecifically, possesses a four- to six-word vocabulary, identifies a body part, uses two-word sentences, and uses pronouns.

A "basal age" occurs when the child passes all items at two conservative age levels; the "ceiling" is the item last passed preceding two higher levels that do not contain any further passes. Performance between ages is interpolated: if a toddler passed all items at 18 months and one of the three items in the 21-month age grouping (with no further passes), the CLAMS age-equivalent would be 19 months (18 + 1). A quotient is derived by dividing the CLAMS age-equivalent by the child's chronological age.

Correlations with the Bayley Scales of Infant Development range from $r = 0.64$ to 0.79 in at-risk populations, although a ratio quotient was devised from the BSID in these comparisons.[32] In general, children scored approximately 10 points higher on the CLAMS than on the Bayley. Reported sensitivity and specificity values are 0.66 and 0.79, respectively (using the BSID as the relative "gold standard").

The CLAMS can be a useful gross screening instrument, however, caution should be exercised because of the ratio quotient. Moreover, primary reliance on parental reports potentially could be problematic. The utility of the scale for children under 12 months of age requires further investigation.

3.10. SUMMARY

It is obvious that speech and language function are extremely important, as language is the primary means by which a child develops social and interpersonal relationships. Moreover, language is the major vehicle for instruction and learning. In view of these risks, primary-care physicians must be aware of early signs of language delay.[6] The assumption should *not* be made that children under 4 years of age who have language delays will catch up automatically. This oversimplification is dangerous,[6] and language delays can be identified as early as age 2 years.[12,13]

The physician should be cognizant that language develops very rapidly over the first 3 years, with a particularly sensitive period occurring between 9 and 24 months. It is estimated that 80% of all language is learned during these first 3 years and that the bulk of a child's understanding of grammar, syntax, and pronunciation is achieved by 3 to 5 years.[8,33,34] Early detection of language problems is therefore important, because early therapy/intervention is associated with a better long-term prognosis. The older the child, the greater the effort required to correct deficits (if they can be corrected).[35]

3.11. DIAGNOSTIC CLUES

The preceding discussion must be placed in an applied context. Practitioners should be cognizant that the primary factors for underreferral of very young children with suspected language delays are (1) the paucity of adequate assessment instruments and (2) the large degree of variability found in "normal" language development. In reference to the latter issue, the average number of words comprehended by a 12-month-old infant is approximately 85; however, the range is from 9 to 225.[6] Similarly, the mean number of words used expressively by infants at this age is 13, but this number ranges from 0 to 83. At 24 months of age, the average number of words used is 300, but once again the normal range is large, extending from 28 to over 600 words. Nonetheless, proper evaluation of speech–language function is essential.

Clinical judgment and parental report have been reported to be useful in the detection of speech–language impairment.[36] In a study of 157 families, 72% of children whose speech–language screening yielded positive results had parents who raised concerns about their child's development in this area. Of those children whose speech–language screening was negative, 83% had parents who did not raise concerns. However, almost twice as many parents had concerns as had children with speech–language delays, suggesting a very high rate of overreferral. These findings suggest that the primary-care physician should incorporate parental report into clinical decision making regarding language function, perhaps considering it as a "prescreening" mechanism.

A clinical decision tree for evaluation of suspected speech–language delays is found in Figure 3.3. If speech–language concerns are raised by parents, further evaluation is necessary. A hearing evaluation should be performed (particularly if there is a history of recurrent ear infections). If

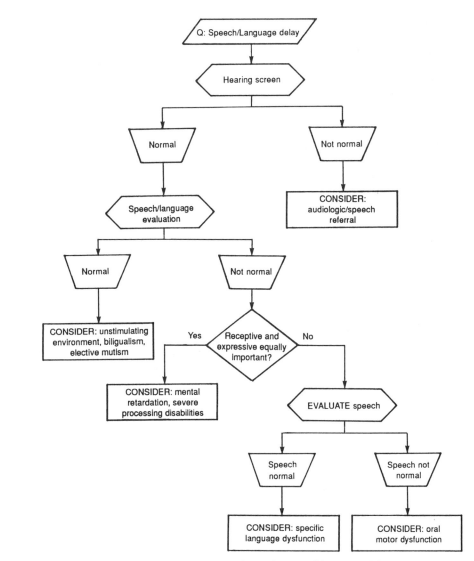

FIGURE 3.3. Decision tree for evaluation of language delay.

hearing problems are identified, referral to an audiologist or speech therapist is recommended. If the hearing evaluation is normal, further screening/assessment of speech–language function is necessary (left side of decision tree).

If the assessment results are negative, other possibilities for language problems should be considered, such as an understimulating environment, bilingualism, or elective mutism. However, if evaluation results are positive, mental retardation, oral-motor problems, or specific language disorders must be considered, depending on the profile of results (see Figure 3.3). In particular, the practitioner must consider the relationship between expressive and receptive language function. If both are equally impaired, the likelihood increases of mental retardation or a severe processing disorder. A marked discrepancy between expressive and receptive language necessitates a more in-depth speech evaluation.

Once again, the primary-care physician can administer these tests, have ancillary office professionals perform this screening, or refer to other professionals for further testing. Regardless of which of these alternatives is selected, early identification of speech–language problems is mandatory.

ACKNOWLEDGMENTS

A special thanks is extended to Margaret Cullen, M.A., slp/ccc, Certified Speech/Language pathologist, Memorial Medical Center, Springfield, IL, and Adjunct Instructor, Department of Pediatrics, Southern Illinois University School of Medicine, for her thoughtful comments on this chapter.

REFERENCES

1. Howlin, P., and Kendall, L., 1991, Assessing children with language tests—which test to use? *J. Dis. Commun.* **26:**355–367.
2. Strominger, A. Z., and Bashir, A. S., 1977, A nine-year follow-up of language impaired children, Paper presented to the American Speech and Hearing Association, Chicago, November.
3. Aram, D. M.,Ekelman, B. L., and Nation, J. E., 1984, Preschoolers with language disorders: 10 years later, *J. Speech Hearing Res.* **27:**232–244.
4. Padgett, S. Y., 1988, Speech- and language-impaired three and four year olds: A five year follow-up study, in: *Preschool Prevention of Reading Failure* (R. L. Masland and M. W. Masland, eds.), pp. 52–77, York Press, Parkton, MD.
5. Scarborough H. S., and Dobrich, W., 1990, Development of children with early language delay, *J. Speech Hearing Res.* **33:**70–83.

6. Thal, E., and Bates, E., 1989, Language and communication in early childhood, *Pediatr. Ann.* **18:**299–305.
7. Locke, J. L., 1992, Thirty years of research on developmental neurolinguistics, *Pediatr. Neurol.* **8:**245–250.
8. Schwartz, A. H., and Murphy, M. W., 1975, Cues for screening language disorders in preschool children, *Pediatrics* **55:**717–722.
9. Perkins, W. H., 1971, *Speech Pathology: An Applied Behavioral Science*, C. V. Mosby, St. Louis.
10. McCauley, R., and Swisher, L., 1984, Psychometric review of language and articulation tests for preschool children. *J. Speech Hearing Dis.* **49:**338–348.
11. Bishop, D., and Edmundson, A., 1987, Language impaired 4-year-olds: Distinguishing transient from persistent impairment, *J. Speech Hearing Dis.* **52:**156–173.
12. Rescorla, L., 1989, The language development survey: A screening tool for delayed language in toddlers, *J. Speech Hearing Dis.* **82:**218–227.
13. Capute, A., Palmer, F., Shapiro, B., et al., 1986, Clinical linguistic and auditory milestone scale: Prediction of cognition in infancy, *Dev. Med. Child. Neurol.* **28:**762–771.
14. Dunn, L. M., and Dunn, L. M., 1981, *Peabody Picture Vocabulary Test-R*, American Guidance Service, Circle Pines, MN.
15. Bracken, B. A., Prasse, D. P., and McCallum, R. S., 1984, Peabody Picture Vocabulary Test-Revised: An appraisal and review, *School Psychol. Rev.* **13:**49–60.
16. Coplan, J., 1987, *Early Language Milestone Scale*, Pro-ED, Inc., Austin, TX.
17. Coplan, J., Gleason, J. R., Ryan, R., Burke, M. G., and Williams, M. L., 1982, Validation of an early language milestone scale in a high-risk population, *Pediatrics* **70:**677–683.
18. Borowitz, K. C., and Glascoe, F. P., 1986, Sensitivity of the Denver Developmental Screening Test in speech and language screening, *Pediatrics* **78:**1075–1078.
19. Walker, D., Gugenheim, S., Downs, M. P., and Northern, J. L., 1989, Early Language Milestone Scale and language screening of young children, *Pediatrics* **83:**284–288.
20. Satish, M., McQuiston, S., Dennler, J., Mueller, P., et al., 1988, Developmental testing II. Correlation of multiple Early Language Milestone (ELM) with Bayley, *Pediatr. Res.* **23:**455A.
21. Coplan, J., and Gleason, J. R., 1990, Quantifying language development from birth to 3 years using the Early Language Milestone Scale, *Pediatrics* **86:**963–971.
22. Robert Wood Johnson Foundation and University of Colorado Health Sciences Center, 1986, *Guidelines for Hearing and Language Screening of Young Children in Physician's Offices*, University of Colorado Health Sciences Center, Denver.
23. Coplan, J., and Gleason, J. R., 1988, Unclear speech: Recognition and significance of unintelligible speech in preschool children, *Pediatrics* **82:**447–452.
24. Zimmerman, I. L., Steiner, V. G., and Pond, R. E., 1979, *Preschool Language Scale*, Charles E. Merrill, Columbus, OH.
25. Zimmerman, I. L., Steiner, V. G., and Pond, R. E., 1992, *Preschool Language Scale-3*, The Psychological Corporation, San Antonio.
26. Boehm, A. E., 1986, *Boehm Test of Basic Concepts-Revised*, The Psychological Corporation, New York.
27. Boehm, A. E., 1986, *Boehm Test of Basic Concepts—Preschool Version*, The Psychological Corporation, San Antonio.
28. Bzoch, K. R., and League, R., 1970, *Receptive-Expressive Emergent Language Scale (REEL Scale)*, University Park Press, Baltimore.
29. Fudala, J. B., 1974, *Arizona Articulation Proficiency Scale-Revised*, Western Psychological Services, Los Angeles.
30. Fudala, J. B., and Reynolds, W. M., 1986, *Arizona Articulation Proficiency Scale*, ed. 2, Western Psychological, Los Angeles.

31. Lee, L. L., 1971, *Northwestern Syntax Screening Test*, Northwestern University Press, Evanston, IL.
32. Capute, A. J., Shapiro, B. K., Wachtel, R. C., Gunther, V. A., and Palmer, F. B., 1986, The Clinical Linguistic and Auditory Milestone Scale (CLAMS), *Am. J. Dis. Child.* **140:** 694–698.
33. Lenneberg, E. H., 1967, *Biological Foundations of Language*. John Wiley & Sons, New York.
34. McNeill, D., 1970, *The Acquisition of Language: The Study of Developmental Psycholinguistics*, Harper & Row, New York.
35. Denhoff, E., 1981, Current status of infant stimulation or enrichment programs for children with developmental disabilities, *Pediatrics* **67:**32–37.
36. Glasco, F. P., 1991, Can clinical judgement detect children with speech–language problems? *Pediatrics* **87:**317–322.

4 ❉ Evaluation of Behavioral/Adaptive Functioning

4.1. INTRODUCTION

Behavioral/adaptive function is another area that should be considered in the evaluation of a child with suspected developmental delay. The American Association on Mental Deficiency (AAMD) defines adaptive behavior as "the effectiveness with which the individual meets the standards of personal independence and social responsibility"[1] (p. 1). Adaptive behavior is both age and culture specific and typically includes independent functioning, social responsibility, and cognitive development.[1] Sensorimotor, communication, and self-help skills are measured in the preschool period. At older ages, practical application of academic skills and appropriate interpersonal function can be assessed. Public Law 94-142 and the AAMD both stipulate that deficits in adaptive behavior and intelligence must be substantiated before an individual is classified as "mentally retarded." A more comprehensive overview of adaptive behavior can be found in a 1987 special issue of the *Journal of Special Education*.[2]

Five instruments have been selected for discussion in this section: (1) the Vineland Adaptive Behavior Scales,[3] (2) the Preschool Attainment Record,[4] (3) the Minnesota Child Development Inventory,[5] (4) the Scales of Independent Behavior,[6] and (5) the AAMD Adaptive Behavior Scale—School Edition.[7] Other popular measures of adaptive behavior that are not reviewed in detail include the Comprehensive Test of Adaptive Behavior[8] (ages 5–60 years), the Normative Adaptive Behavior Checklist[9] (infancy–21 years), and the Inventory for Client and Agency Planning[10] (infancy–40+ years). In general, there is a need to supplement formal developmental assessments with psychometrically sound parent-report inventories.

4.2. VINELAND ADAPTIVE BEHAVIOR SCALES

The Vineland Adaptive Behavior Scales[3] (VABS) is one of the most frequently used measures of adaptive functioning. The origins of this test instrument can be found in the Vineland Social Maturity Scale (VSMS),[11,12] first published in 1953 and containing 117 items, applicable from birth to maturity. The VSMS was normed by door-to-door interviewing of 620 individuals utilizing the measurement of skills such as self-help, dressing, eating, locomotion, occupation, communication, self-direction, and socialization. Although it was useful in the assessment of severely and profoundly retarded individuals, there were significant problems with reliability and validity.

There are three editions of the current VABS: the Interview Edition Survey Form, the Interview Edition Expanded Form, and the Classroom Edition. The forms differ in the number of test items and administration time (from 20 to 60 min). The Survey Form, which is most practical for use by practitioners, consists of 297 items, answered by the parent/caregiver. Behavioral descriptions are presented to the parent, who is required to respond "yes, usually" (2 points), "sometimes or partially" (1 point), or "no, never" (0 points). All of the test items are not presented at each age. The Expanded Form contains 577 items. The Classroom Edition has 244 items and is completed by the teacher. Four adaptive behavior domains are evaluated: skills in (1) communication (gestures, number of words in vocabulary, speaks in full sentences), (2) daily living (drinks from cup, puts shoes on, is toilet trained), (3) socialization (plays interactive games, imitates adult phrases, says "please"), and (4) motor function (transfers objects, jumps, walks down stairs) are assessed. In addition, maladaptive behaviors (tics, extreme anxiety, runs away, has temper tantrums) are documented.

A standard score (M = 100, SD = 15) as well as percentile ranks, stanines, adaptive levels, and age equivalents in each of these areas or "domains" is obtained. There are additional breakdowns of specific functional areas within each of the four domains. A moderately low adaptive level is one to two standard deviations below average; a low adaptive level is two standard deviations below average. When the VABS is administered, a basal age is established when seven "yes, usually" responses to items are obtained; the ceiling is seven "no, never" responses. The motor scale scores are applicable up to age 6 years, but the motor function domain items can be administered to older, delayed children, with age equivalents being obtained (see Figure 4.1).

The time spent in administration varies, depending on the chronological and developmental age of the child. Reliability of parent or caretaker

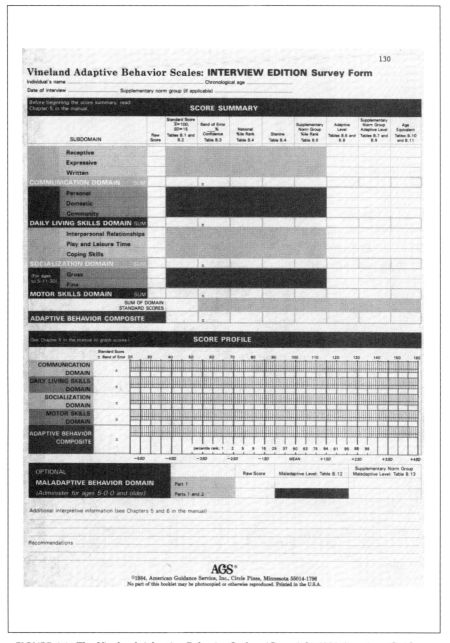

FIGURE 4.1. The Vineland Adaptive Behavior Scales. (Copyright 1984 American Guidance Service, Inc., 4201 Woodland Road, Circle Pines, Minnesota 55014-1796. All rights reserved.)

report is also variable; nonetheless, the VABS is very helpful in the total evaluation of the child. As mentioned previously, measurements of this type are essential in the assessment of mental retardation, because both IQ estimates and measures of adaptive functioning are necessary to make this diagnosis. As was indicated above, the VABS probably is the measure of adaptive functioning used most frequently in clinical practice.

4.3. PRESCHOOL ATTAINMENT RECORD

The Preschool Attainment Record[4] (PAR) is a 112-item survey instrument applicable to children from birth to $7\frac{1}{2}$ years. The PAR is an extension of the Vineland Social Maturity Scale,[12] and it enables evaluation of physical, social, and intellectual functions. The record consists of eight scales that fall into three developmental areas: (1) physical (ambulation and manipulation), (2) social (rapport, communication, responsibility), and (3) intellectual (information, ideation, creativity). One item at each age level is contained in each of the eight scales (to be answered by a parent/caretaker). An item can be scored in three categories: (1) credit (child can perform task), (2) half-credit (doubtful if child can perform task), and (3) no credit (child cannot perform task).

Sample items on the PAR include: names primary colors, reproduces or echoes words or sounds, and stands in place on each foot alternately. An Attainment Age and an Attainment Quotient (calculated by the ratio method) can be obtained. However, use of the ratio method is a weakness of the test instrument (Chapter 1). The PAR correlates with the DDST ($r = 0.89$), the VSMS ($r = 0.88$), and the Gesell ($r = 0.86$); however, the standardization procedures are psychometrically weak. In general, the PAR is particularly useful in children younger than 5 years of age.

4.4. MINNESOTA CHILD DEVELOPMENT INVENTORY

The Minnesota Child Development Inventory[5] (MCDI) was designed for children aged 1 to 6 years. The test contains 320 statements that describe a child's behavior and development. The parent is required to respond to items in eight developmental scales: (1) gross motor, (2) fine motor, (3) expressive language, (4) comprehension (language/conceptual), (5) comprehension (situation), (6) self-help, (7) personal–social, and (8) a general development scale (which contains the most discriminating items from the seven other scales). The instrument takes approximately 30 to 45 min to complete and 15 min or less to score. Prior to 36 months of age, there appears to be greater item sampling for virtually all of the eight scales except for fine motor.[5] Sample items for each of the areas are found in Table 4.1. Caretakers are requested to answer "yes" if the child presently or previously demonstrated the behavior and "no" if the child has never demonstrated the behavior.

The Minnesota Preschool Inventory[13] is designed specifically to assess kindergarten readiness in children aged 4 to 6 years. This scale contains 150 statements from seven developmental areas (similar to the MCDI with the addition of letter recognition and number comprehension) and four adjustment areas (immaturity, hyperactivity, behavioral problems, emotional problems). An abbreviated version of the General Development Scale of the MCDI that is applicable to pediatric practice has also been developed.[14]

Levels of development in each area are categorized as "normal" (≤30% below the child's age level), "delayed" (between 30% and 50% below age level), and "seriously delayed" (>50% below the child's age level). The term "apparently" is utilized when an assigned score may be unreliable because of a limited number of applicable items. Age levels for each of the eight scales also can be obtained. According to the MCDI manual, approximately 2% of the children in the general population would receive a score at the 30% below age level cut-off.

TABLE 4.1. Sample MCDI Items for Each Scale[4]

Gross motor	Situation comprehension
Rolls over from stomach to back	Plays "peek-a-boo"
Stands without support	Opens door by turning knob
Runs	Imitates mother
Hops on one foot	Self-help
Fine motor	Feeds self a cracker or cookie
Claps hands	Pulls off socks
Builds a tower of two or more blocks	Eats with a fork
Draws simple designs	Takes a bath without help
Colors within lines	Personal/social
Expressive language	Plays with other children
Makes sounds like da, ba, ga, ka, ma	Actively refuses to obey
Points	Helps set the table
Says "thank you"	Crosses the street alone
Uses at least ten words	
Language comprehension	
Follows simple instructions	
Identifies at least one color correctly	
Counts to ten	
Tells what an object is made of	

The MCDI scales correspond with results of developmental evalua-tions and can differentiate children who have behavioral problems from those who do not.[15] Correlations with the MSCA are typically significant ($r = 0.60$ and above), as are correlations between the MCDI and, at older ages, the Wechsler Intelligence Scale for Children-Revised full-scale IQs ($r = 0.63$).[17] The MCDI General Development, Language, and Comprehen-sion Scales are the best predictors of later intelligence, academic achieve-ment, adjustment, and social-adaptive function.[17] The motor scales are not as predictive.

A recent investigation of the association between the MCDI and the Bayley Scales in a high-risk infant population indicates that the usefulness of the MCDI in the assessment of at-risk children under 2 years of age is limited by low sensitivity (copositivity).[18] Specificity is adequate, suggest-ing that few "normal" infants would be diagnosed incorrectly; however, the high underreferral rate of "not normal" infants is a cause for concern.

The MCDI is scored with templates or is machine-scored with an interpretive summary provided. This summary is particularly helpful for the primary-care physician because it indicates whether development is normal or delayed in specific areas. Although emphasized as a develop-mental screening instrument, the data from the comprehension, self-help, and personal–social scales are useful in the assessment of the behavioral/adaptive realm. Basically, questionnaires of this type afford information about the child's functioning in his/her natural environment.

4.5. SCALES OF INDEPENDENT BEHAVIOR

The Scales of Independent Behavior[6] (SIB), normed on 1500 individ-uals, was designed "to assess skills needed to function independently in home, social, and community settings"[6] (p. 5). It is intended for ages infancy through adulthood and is administered individually by use of a structured interview that takes approximately 45 to 60 min. There are three forms of the SIB: (1) the full SIB, (2) the Short Form, and (3) the Early Development Scale. The Broad Independence Scale of the full SIB consists of four clusters: (1) motor skills (gross and fine motor), (2) social interaction and communication skills (social interaction, language comprehension, language expression), (3) personal living skills (eating, toileting, dressing, personal self-care, domestic skills), and (4) community living skills (time and punctuality, money, work skills, home/community orientation). A Problem Behaviors Scale that enables assessment of eight problem behav-ior areas also is provided [internalized maladaptive (e.g., hurtful to self), asocial, and externalized (e.g., hurtful to others)].

A short form consisting of 32 items selected from all 14 subscales is also available for quick screening. This version takes approximately 10 to 15 min to administer.

Primary-care physicians generally are most interested in the Early Development Scale, which is applicable from birth to $2\frac{1}{2}$ years of age. This scale, which contains 32 items, can also be used with older children whose developmental levels are $2\frac{1}{2}$ years or below. The Early Development Scale requires only approximately 10 to 15 min to administer.

Items are scored on a 0 to 3 scale: "0" for "never or rarely, even if asked," or does less than 5% of the time; "1" for "does, but not well, may need to be asked" or does 25% of the time; "2" for "does fairly well, may need to be asked" or does 75% of the time; and "3" for "does very well, always or almost always, without being asked."[18] The basal level is established when all four items on a page are scored "3"; the ceiling is four consecutive "0" scorings.

On the Early Development Scale, areas assessed include responsiveness to persons (looks, reaches, turns head when name is called), eating (soft foods, crackers, drinks without spilling), peer interactions (plays simple games, group games), dressing (removes socks, pants, underwear), language (uses ten words, follows directions), object permanency, and fine and gross motor skills (transfers, sits, stands alone).

Percentiles, standard scores (M = 100, SD = 15), age equivalents, and stanines are obtained. A Relative Performance Index (RPI) is used for interpretive purposes on the SIB.[19] Similar to the Snellen visual acuity method (i.e., 20/20), the RPI has 90 as a constant denominator. Therefore, an RPI of 70/90 indicates that the child would be predicted to achieve a 70% success level on tasks that peers would perform at a 90% success level; 100/90 would indicate an above-average level of performance.

The SIB is well standardized, reliable, and valid.[19,20] It is statistically linked to the Woodcock Johnson Psychoeducational Battery cognitive and academic scores, and this is an advantage. A computerized scoring program is also available.

4.6. INVENTORY FOR CLIENT AND AGENCY PLANNING

Of note is that the previously mentioned Inventory for Client and Agency Planning[10] (ICAP) contains 77 adaptive behavior items (arranged into four domains: motor skills, social and communication skills, personal living skills, community living skills) that were selected from the SIB. Because the ICAP can be given by a variety of professionals and administration time is relatively short (20 min), this instrument is particularly attractive for social workers, school psychologists, therapists, and case managers.

4.7. AAMD ADAPTIVE BEHAVIOR SCALE

The Adaptive Behavior Scale (ABS) comes in two versions: (1) the ABS School Edition (for children ages 3–17 years) and (2) a version for handicapped populations. Both versions are comprised of two parts: Part I assesses adaptive behavior (personal independence and development), whereas Part II involves behavior related to emotional adjustment.

Part I assesses nine domains (see Table 4.2), with the caretaker selecting the descriptor that best applies to the child. For example, in the eating subdomain, the "drinking" item ranges from "drinks without spilling" (score of 3) to "does not drink from cup or glass unassisted" (score of 0). Scores can be collapsed into three broad factors: (1) Personal Self-Sufficiency, (2) Community Self-Sufficiency, and (3) Personal–Social Responsibility. Each is reported in a standard score format. An overall composite score derived from these three factors can be calculated. The child's performance may be compared to three normative samples: (1) children in regular classes, (2) those in classes for children with mild mental retardation (educable mentally retarded; EMH), and (3) children with more severe mental retardation (trainable mentally retarded; TMH). Therefore, it can be determined which group of children has adaptive skills most like those under consideration.

The ABS recently has been revised and renamed the AAMR Adaptive Behavior Scales-School.[19] Part I contains nine behavior domains (see Table 4.2), whereas Part II contains content related to social maladaptation (e.g., violent and antisocial behavior, stereotyped and hyperactive behavior, withdrawal). Domain raw scores are converted to standard scores (M = 10,

---

TABLE 4.2. Behavior Domains of AAMR Adaptive Behavior Scales—School[21]

1. *Independent functioning*: eating, toilet training, appearance, clothing, dressing/undressing, utilizing public transportation
2. *Physical development*: sensory and motor abilities
3. *Economic activity*: ability to manage financial affairs, consumer issues
4. *Numbers and time*: basic mathematics competencies
5. *Prevocational/vocational*: job and school performance
6. *Responsibility*: responsibility for actions, duties, and belongings
7. *Self-direction*: active or passive life-style
8. *Socialization*: ability to interact with others

SD = 3) and percentiles. Factor raw scores generate quotients (M = 100, SD = 15) and percentiles.

4.8. SUMMARY

The AAMD defines mental retardation as follows: "Mental retardation refers to significantly subaverage general intellectual functioning existing concurrently with deficits in adaptive behavior and manifested during the developmental period"[1] (p. 11). However, until fairly recently, measurement of adaptive behavior was considered incidental rather than essential. Assessment of this area is very important because of (1) the weight afforded to both adaptive and cognitive function in the evaluation of developmental delay and (2) the documented relationship between adaptive function and later-life adjustment.

Measures of adaptive function are particularly useful in program planning/placement, appraising developmental gains, and evaluating children with mild mental retardation. Screening instruments of adaptive function such as the Scales of Independent Behavior Short Form,[6] the SIB Early Development Scale,[6] or the Inventory for Client and Agency Planning[10] (ICAP) can easily be administered by office personnel who have had some training.

REFERENCES

1. Grossman, H. J. (ed.), 1983, *Classification in Mental Retardation*, American Association on Mental Deficiency, Washington, DC.
2. Kamphaus, R. W., 1987, Adaptive behavior (special issue), *J. Spec.Ed.* **21**.
3. Sparrow, S. S., Bulla, D. A., and Cicchetti, D. V., 1984, *Vineland Adaptive Behavior Scales*, American Guidance Service, Circle Pines, MN.
4. Doll, E. A., 1966, *PAR, Preschool Attainment Record, Research Edition Manual*, American Guidance Service, Circle Pines, MN.
5. Ireton, H., and Thwing, E., 1974, *Manual for the Minnesota Child Development Inventory*, Behavioral Science Systems, Minneapolis.
6. Bruininks, R. H., Woodcock, R. W., Weatherman, R. F., and Hill, B. K., 1984, *Scales of Independent Behavior*, DLM Teaching Resources, Allen, TX.
7. Lambert, N., Windmiller, M., Tharinger, D., and Cole, L., 1981, *AAMD Adaptive Behavior Scale-School Edition*, American Association on Mental Deficiency, Washington, DC.
8. Adams, G. L., 1984, *Comprehensive Test of Adaptive Behavior*, Psychological Corporation, San Antonio, TX.
9. Adams, G. L., 1984, *Normative Adaptive Behavior Checklist*, Psychological Corporation, San Antonio, TX.
10. Bruininks, R. H., Hill, B. K., Weatherman, R. F., and Woodcock, R. W., 1986, *Inventory for Client and Agency Planning*, DLM Teaching Resources, Allen, TX.

11. Doll, E. A., 1953, Vineland Social Maturity Scale, in: *Contributions Toward Medical Psychology: Theory and Psychodiagnostic Methods*, Volume 2 (A. Weider, ed.), Ronald Press, New York.
12. Doll, E. A., 1965, *Vineland Social Maturity Scale*, American Guidance Service, Circle Pines, MN.
13. Ireton, H., and Thwing, E., 1979, *Manual for the Minnesota Preschool Inventory*, Behavioral Science Systems, Minneapolis.
14. Sturner, R. A., Funk, S. G., Thomas, P. D., and Green, J. A., 1982, An adaptation of the Minnesota Child Development Inventory for preschool developmental screening, *J. Pediatr. Psychol.* **7:**295–306.
15. Garity, L. I., and Servos, A. B., 1978, Comparison of measures of adaptive behaviors in preschool children, *J. Consult. Clin. Psychol.* **46:**288–293.
16. Gottfried, A. W., Guerin, D., Spencer, J. E., and Meyer, C., 1984, Validity of Minnesota Child Development Inventory in screening young children's developmental status, *J. Pediatr. Psychol.* **9:**219–230.
17. Guerin, D., and Gottfried, A. W., 1987, Minnesota Child Development Inventories: Predictors of intelligence, achievement, and adaptability, *J. Pediatr. Psychol.* **12:**595–609.
18. Kopparthi, R., McDermott, C., and Sheftel, D., 1991, The Minnesota Child Development Inventory: Validity and reliability for assessing development in infancy, *J. Dev. Behav. Pediatr.* **12:**217–222.
19. Harrington, R. G., 1986, Scales of Independent Behavior, in: *Test Critiques*, Volume III (D. J. Keyser and R. C. Sweetland, eds.), Test Corporation of America, Kansas City, MO, pp. 551–563.
20. Cummings, J. A., and Simon, M. S., 1988, Test review: Scales of Independent Behavior: Woodcock–Johnson Psycho-Educational Battery—Part Four, *J. Psychoed. Assess.* **6:**315–320.
21. Nihara, K., Lambert, N., and Leland, H., 1992, *AAMR Adaptive Behavior Scales—School*, ed. 2, Pro-Ed, Austin, TX.

5 ❊ Summary of Developmental Assessment

5.1. INTRODUCTION

When infants and young children are referred for evaluation of a suspected developmental disorder, the physician must consider a variety of intrinsic and extrinsic factors. An appreciation of "normal" behavior and development is essential in order to identify that which is "abnormal."

In the United States, the majority of states have designated Departments of Public Health as the lead agency under PL 99-457. Therefore, primary-care physicians have a critical role in the early identification of young handicapped children, and this has resulted in the publication of numerous reviews of available screening tests.[1] The passage of federal and state mandates in the form of PL 99-457 and the IDEA amendments (see Chapter 2) has prompted many professional organizations to publish formal policy statements regarding early childhood assessment, intervention, and training.[2] These include the National Association of School Psychologists[3] (NASP), The Council for Exceptional Children-Division for Early Childhood[4] (DEC), and the American Speech and Hearing Association[5] (ASHA).

Assessment for early intervention requires collaborative teamwork, converging information, and a developmental perspective (versus a traditional psychometric approach); it must be intervention based (i.e., have a direct link to programming) and family directed[2] as well. Physicians will need to redefine their role within these guidelines.

The physician's role in the management of suspected developmental delays involves (1) performing routine developmental screening and surveillance, (2) discussion of normal developmental variations with parents and professionals, (3) explaining test results to parents, (4) acknowledging parental concerns, (5) providing secondary-level assessment of potential developmental dysfunctions or referring to other professionals for more detailed assessment, and (6) facilitating management interventions.

5.2. RECOMMENDED PROTOCOL FOR EARLY DEVELOPMENTAL SCREEN/ASSESSMENT

The wide variety of developmental assessment inventories that currently are available makes it difficult for the primary-care physician to select one protocol that is feasible for routine surveillance. Many instruments are not practical for office use because of time constraints and/or the level of training required for meaningful administration. A suggested protocol for primary-level screening and subsequent, more detailed assessment will be reviewed in the discussion to follow. It is assumed that a routine medical evaluation will be undertaken at each time period as well.

At 2 to 4 months, the primary-care physician should routinely perform a general screening of the infant's vision, hearing, and muscle tone. General development can be screened with the 0- to 9-month form of the revised Prescreening Developmental Questionnaire[6] (R-PDQ) and/or the DDST-II,[7] and neuromotor function with the Milani-Comparetti–Gidoni[8] (MCG). The Bayley Infant Neurodevelopmental Screen (BINS)—3-Month Version[9] allows for evaluation of posture, tone, movement, and development level and is recommended as a general brief assessment at this age. If concerns are raised about the child's functioning in these areas, more detailed assessment is necessary.

At 6 months, the R-PDQ[6] and DDST-II[7] or BINS—6 Months[9] similarly may be used to evaluate global development. Language function can be screened with the Early Language Milestone Scale[10] (ELMS) or the Clinical Linguistic and Auditory Milestone Scale[11] (CLAMS). The Milani-Comparetti–Gidoni again is useful for neuromotor screening. The short form of the Scales of Independent Behavior (SIB), the SIB Early Development Scale,[12] and the Inventory for Client and Agency Planning[13] (ICAP) are useful in assessing adaptive function. However, because this area of development becomes more significant with advancing age, screening of adaptive function can be postponed if necessary until 1 to 2 years of age. This protocol also can be applied at 12 and 24 months (using the BINS—12, —18, or —24 Months[9]). The ELMS or CLAMS and the DDST-II can be administered at 3 years of age. If questions arise concerning behavioral/adaptive development, temperament questionnaires[14,15] and the computer-scored Minnesota Child Development Inventory (MCDI) are appropriate inventories.

More detailed secondary-level assessment, which may also be administered in an office setting, includes (1) the Gesell[17] or the Battelle Screening Test[18] for evaluation of global development, (2) the Peabody Picture Vocabulary Test-R[19] or the Receptive–Expressive Emergent Language Scale (REEL)[20] for language, and (3) the Preschool Attainment Record[21] (PAR) or the SIB Early Development Scale[12] for assessment of behavioral/adaptive function.

The Bayley Scales[22] (or Bayley II), Battelle Developmental Inventory,[18] McCarthy Scales of Children's Abilities,[23] or the Differential Ability Scales[24] can be used for more in-depth assessment of cognitive and global development. However, these instruments will probably need to be administered by specially trained professionals. Similarly, the Preschool Language Scale-3[25] or the Boehm Test of Basic Concepts[26] may be used to provide more detailed assessment of language. The Vineland Adaptive Behavior Scales[27] or Scales of Independent Behavior[12] can provide a good evaluation of adaptive functioning.

5.3. DECISION TREE FOR SUSPECTED DEVELOPMENTAL DELAY

As was indicated previously, when a parent or the practitioner suspects developmental delays, three domains of function must be considered: cognitive/motor, language, and adaptive functioning. Practitioners should be aware that categorization of tests into cognitive/motor, language, and adaptive groupings is somewhat artificial, as many tests overlap two or even three groupings. Nonetheless, it is advisable to use a general developmental test and supplement this with tests that measure more specific areas of function. Application of the recommended protocol in a procedural decision tree is found in Figure 5.1.

A general developmental screening or brief assessment instrument such as the Bayley Infant Neurodevelopmental Screen[9] (BINS), Denver II,[7] or the Battelle Screening Inventory[18] should be used in the first step. If the results are negative and the practitioner is fairly confident that these results are valid, then continued developmental surveillance is recommended, which includes frequent parental ratings (right side of decision tree). If, however, findings from the initial screening/brief assessment are positive, more detailed assessment, using an instrument such as the Bayley Scales or Bayley II, is necessary. If these test results are not indicative of delays, surveillance and retesting in 3 to 6 months are recommended, particularly because the likelihood of obtaining a positive finding with a screening instrument and a negative result with more detailed assessment is low. The profile of a positive finding must be evaluated in more detail; if delays are

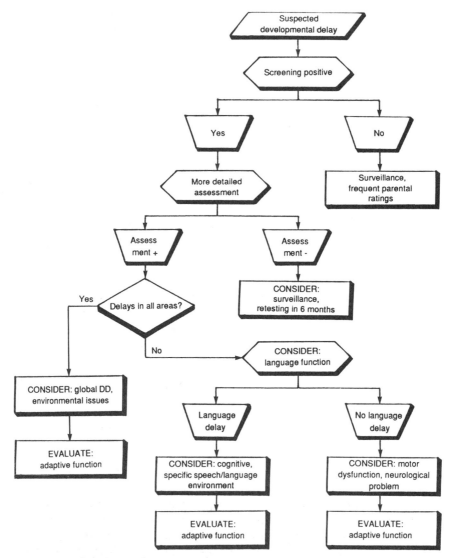

FIGURE 5.1. Decision tree for suspected developmental delay.

found in all areas, compromised development is likely, although environmental aspects and levels of adaptive function must be clarified (left side of decision tree). If delays do not extend to all domains, then language function must be evaluated in detail with tests such as the Early Language Milestone Scale[10] (ELMS-2), Peabody Picture Vocabulary Test[19] (PPVT-R), or the Preschool Language Scale-3 (PLS-3) (bottommost portion of decision tree). Obviously, adaptive function must also be assessed in each of these cases as well.

5.4. EXPLAINING TEST RESULTS

The primary-care physician frequently will be required to explain test results obtained from screening or assessment of a young patient or from data obtained by other professionals. This will involve review of normal developmental variations and acknowledgment of parental concerns. Familiarity with test instruments and knowledge of their limitations in regard to sensitivity, specificity, and predictive validity are necessary.

When abnormal developmental functions are suspected or defined, a balance must be struck between minimizing concerns and excessively alarming parents. It often is helpful initially to ask parents about their thoughts concerning the child's level of development, particularly as it compares to that of other children his or her age. This technique also enables the practitioner to gauge how best to present his or her findings. The concept that the child "will tell us about his/her development as it unfolds" is a useful approach. Physicians are advised to avoid telling parents that their child "will grow out of it." Too often children do not outgrow developmental/behavioral problems. This cliche initially is used to suppress anger from the parents. However, in the long term it may not only engender even more exaggerated anger, but it literally wastes time that could have been spent in early-intervention programs.

Joining with parents in genuinely wanting the "best" for their child (the physician's patient) is clearly acknowledged. It should be clearly established that the clinician does not have an emotional investment in finding developmental/behavioral delays and would be delighted if proven wrong by significant improvement in the child's developmental status. Similarly, if a significant delay is detected (e.g., developmental quotient ≥ 2 SD below average), informing parents that they will probably encounter terms such as "mental retardation" or "cerebral palsy" is appropriate. It is suggested that the term "mental retardation" be reserved for children over 2 years of age; "developmental delay" (a noncategorical term) can be used for younger children and infants.

A question typically asked by parents who have been informed about their child's developmental delay(s) usually relates to long-term educational and vocational goals. Specific predictions about long-term outcomes should be avoided, except to comment that there is a strong probability that special educational interventions will be required, but the type or amount is not known at this time. In the case of mild delays, offering the suggestion that the child will most likely be a productive member of society is appropriate. Explanations regarding the range of special educational services (e.g., learning disability pull-out programs to self-contained TMH classes) or vocational abilities (living independently to group homes) are often helpful to parents.

A major pitfall frequently encountered when one is explaining developmental delays to parents involves the concept of "age equivalents" (see Chapter 1). For example, in the case of a 12-month-old infant functioning at a 6-month age level on the Bayley Scales, there is an obvious 6-month delay. Parents may assume, however, that the 6-month lag is fixed, meaning that at 24 months, the child would be functioning at an 18-month level. The concept of a "ratio" should be emphasized; namely, 6 months:12 months equals a development rate of one-half. Therefore, at 24 months, one would expect the child's function to be at a 12-month level. Rate of development can be explained to parents using a diagram (see Figure 5.2, where line A represents "average"—avoid "normal"—development; the rate of development in the child with the current 6-month delay is indicated by line B; lines C and D—dashed—represent future possibilities as to the child's developmental slope or progress). Suggesting that the child's subsequent developmental level would very likely fall between B and C is valid in conjunction with an opinion that there is little possibility that the subsequent slope would approach line A. The current developmental assessment should be considered a "snapshot," and the need for a "moving picture" (serial evaluations) should be emphasized. That some developmental gains will occur generally may be guaranteed; however, the type and degree cannot be predicted. Finally, it is helpful to request that the parents recount what they have been told about the test results. This offers an opportunity to explore misconceptions and to provide clarifications when necessary.

5.5. SELF-MONITORING

Primary-care physicians must be careful to monitor their subjective impressions of their patients' development. Several recent studies have indicated that approximately 50% of children with developmental delays

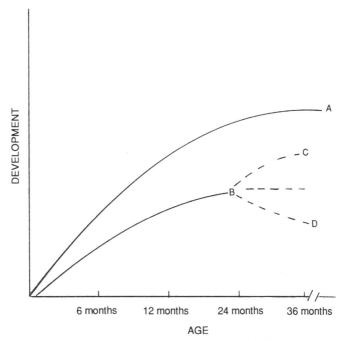

FIGURE 5.2. Hypothetical diagram to explain developmental delay. Line A represents "average" development; Line B is a given child's developmental level. The dashed lines represent possible subsequent developmental courses.

are detected prior to school entrance.[28] Pediatricians have been found to underestimate intelligence in chronically ill children and to overestimate intelligence in children with documented mental retardation. There also is a tendency to overestimate IQ in chronically ill children whom the practitioner knows well.[29] Moreover, when parents raise concerns about their child's development, pediatricians are more likely to be accurate in their estimation of the child's developmental levels.[30]

Time available to address developmental concerns in routine office practice and reimbursement for diagnosis and treatment are limited. This affects how the practitioner deals with developmental and behavioral issues. In addition, the physician's "mind set" will influence his/her ability to detect developmental problems. For example, if the practitioner believes that developmental problems routinely are severe or always extend across multiple developmental functions (e.g., severe mental retardation coupled with cerebral palsy), the likelihood is decreased that mild or more circumscribed deficits will be detected. Similarly, if the practitioner perceives that such problems are infrequent, then the likelihood of identifying them when they do occur is decreased. As was indicated earlier (Chapter 2), reliance on attainment of motor milestones as an indication of overall developmental progress can be misleading, as is the tendency to discount the possibility of later developmental delay if early evaluations suggest "normal" developmental function. Moreover, a broad range of possibilities for delays must be considered and evaluated. The physician's preconceived notions and biases about the prevalence and types of developmental delays, level of confidence, and understanding of the etiologies of developmental disorders (e.g., low Apgar scores do not necessarily predict compromised developmental outcome) must be self-monitored in a continuous fashion.

5.6. PROBLEM CASES

The differential diagnosis by a primary-care physician in the evaluation of "suspected developmental delay" should include (1) mental retardation, (2) emerging learning disability, (3) language dysfunction, (4) environmental influences, or (5) a combination of contributing factors. In the following hypothetical cases, a 2- to 3-year-old child was referred because of suspected developmental delay; vision and hearing were within normal limits, and no gross neurological dysfunction was apparent. General health was good. The evaluation instruments described in the preceding chapters were utilized to determine whether a potential delay of greater than one standard deviation below average (indicated by a "+") was found in the developmental, language, or behavioral/adaptive areas (see Table 5.1).

- *Case 1.* Delays are found in all areas, suggesting global or pervasive deficits. Given the uniformity of delays, mental retardation should be a prime consideration.
- *Case 2.* Delays are found in the motor and expressive language realms; however, deficits are not noted in cognitive, receptive language, or adaptive functioning. This profile is suggestive of subtle motor dysfunction such as fine motor and/or oral-motor apraxia.
- *Case 3.* Developmental lags are found in the cognitive, behavioral/ adaptive, and language (receptive and expressive) areas. Motor function is not problematic. Mental retardation and/or a nonstimulating environment should be considered as two potential causes.
- *Case 4.* Delays are detected in the cognitive, expressive, and receptive language areas. This profile is suggestive of the possibility of a specific language dysfunction or environmental deprivation.

TABLE 5.1. Hypothetical Cases Involving Suspected Development Delay

Case	Developmental		Language		Behavioral/ adaptive	Considerations
	Cognitive	Motor	Receptive	Expressive		
1	+[a]	+	+	+	+	Mental retardation
2	−	+	−	+	−	Motor dysfunction/ apraxia
3	+	−	+	+	+	Mental retardation/ environment
4	+	−	+	+	−	Language dysfunction/ environment
5	+	+	+	+	−	Unreliable parental report
6	−	−	−	−	+	Emerging behavioral problem

[a]A + indicates a positive finding (i.e., delay) in a given area.

- *Case 5.* Deficits are evident in all areas except the behavioral/ adaptive realm. In such cases, the practitioner should entertain the possibility of unreliable parental report.
- *Case 6.* Problems are solely restricted to the behavioral/adaptive area. This profile prompts consideration of an emerging behavioral problem versus a developmental delay.

Clearly, if a delay is found in a specific area of development, more detailed evaluation of that area of function is warranted.

REFERENCES

1. Glascoe, F. P., Martin, E. D., and Humphrey, S., 1990, A comparative review of developmental screening tests, *Pediatrics* **86:**547–554.
2. Bagnato, S. J., 1992, Assessment for early intervention: Best practices with young children and families, *Child. Assess. News* **2:**1–8.
3. Bracken, B., Bagnato, S. J., and Barnett, D., 1991, *Early Childhood Assessment: Position Statement*, National Association of School Psychologists, Silver Spring, MD.
4. Neisworth, J. T., and Bagnato, S. J., 1994, Best practice recommendations for early intervention assessment, in: *Best Practices in Early Intervention* (S. Odom, ed.), Council for Exceptional Children, Division for Early Childhood, Reston, VA.
5. American Speech and Hearing Association, 1990, *Guidelines for Practices in Early Interventions*, ASHA, Rockville, MD.
6. Frankenburg, W. K., Fandal, A. W., and Thornton, S. M., 1987, Revision of Denver Prescreening Developmental Questionnaire, *J. Pediatr.* **110:**653–657.
7. Frankenburg, W. K., Dodds, J., Archer, P., Bresnick, B., et al., 1990, *Denver II Screening Manual*, Denver Developmental Materials, Denver.

 8. Stuberg, W. A., Dehne, P. R., Miedaner, J. A., et al., 1987, *Milani-Comparetti Motor Development Screening Test: Test Manual*, Louis Meyer Children's Rehabilitation Institute, University of Nebraska Medical Center, Omaha.
 9. Aylward, G. P., 1992, *The Bayley Infant Neurodevelopmental Screen Standardization Manual*, The Psychological Corporation, San Antonio.
10. Coplan, J., 1987, *The Early Language Milestone Scale Manual*, Modern Education Corporation, Tulsa, OK.
11. Capute, A. J., Shapiro, B. K., Wachtel, R. C., Gunther, V. A., and Palmer, F. B., 1986, The Clinical Linguistic and Auditory Milestone Scale (CLAMS), *Am. J. Dis. Child.* **140:** 694–698.
12. Bruininks, R. H., Woodcock, R. W., Weatherman, R. F., and Hill, B. K., 1984, *Scales of Independent Behavior*, DLM Teaching Resources, Allen, TX.
13. Bruininks, R. H., Hill, B. K., Weatherman, R. F., and Woodcock, R. W., 1986, *Inventory for Client and Agency Planning*, DLM Teaching Resources, Allen, TX.
14. Carey, W. B., and McDevitt, S. C., 1978, Revision of the Infant Temperament Questionnaire, *Pediatrics* **61:**735–739.
15. Fullard, W., McDevitt, S. C., and Carey, W. B., 1984, Assessing temperament in one to three year old children, *J. Pediatr. Psychol.* **9:**205–217.
16. Ireton, H., and Thwing, E., 1972–1974, *Manual for the Minnesota Child Development Inventory*, Behavioral Science Systems, Minneapolis.
17. Knoblock, H., Stevens, F., and Malone, A. F., 1980, *Manual of Developmental Diagnosis*, Harper & Row, New York.
18. Newborg, J., Stock, J. R., Wnek, L., Guidabaldi, J., and Svinicki, J., 1984, *The Battelle Developmental Inventory*, DLM Teaching Resources, Allen, TX.
19. Dunn, L. M., and Dunn, L. M., 1981, *Peabody Picture Vocabulary Test-R*, American Guidance Service, Circle Pines, MN.
20. Bzoch, K. R., and League, R., 1970, *Receptive–Expressive Emergent Language Scale (REEL Scale)*, University Park Press, Baltimore.
21. Doll, E. A., 1966, *PAR, Preschool Attainment Record, Research Edition Manual*, American Guidance Service, Circle Pines, MN.
22. Bayley, N., 1969, *Bayley Scales of Infant Development*, Psychological Corporation, New York.
23. McCarthy, D., 1972, *McCarthy Scales of Children's Abilities*, Psychological Corporation, New York.
24. Elliott, C. D., 1990, *Differential Ability Scales. Introductory and Technical Handbook*, Psychological Corporation, New York.
25. Zimmerman, I. L., Steiner, V. G., and Pond, R. E., 1992, *Preschool Language Scale-3*, The Psychological Corporation, San Antonio.
26. Boehm, A. E., 1986 *Boehm Test of Basic Concepts-Revised*, The Psychological Corporation, San Antonio.
27. Sparrow, S. S., Bulla, D. A., and Cicchetti, D. V., 1984, *Vineland Adaptive Behavior Scales*, American Guidance Service, Circle Pines, MN.
28. Dearlove, J., and Kearney, D., 1990, How good is general practice developmental screening? *Br. Med. J.* **300:**1177–1180.
29. Koroch, B., Cobb, K., and Ashe, B., 1961, Pediatrician's appraisals of patients' intelligence, *Pediatrics* **29:**990–995.
30. Dulcan, M. K., Costello, E. J., Costello, A. J., et al., 1990, The pediatrician as gate keeper to mental health care for children: Do parents' concerns open the gate? *J. Am. Acad. Child Adol. Psychiat.* **29:**453–458.

II ❋ Evaluation of School Performance Problems

6 ❁ Overview of School Performance Problems

6.1. INTRODUCTION

The second most frequent behavioral problem encountered by primary-health-care professionals is the child who presents with impaired learning or school achievement. It has been estimated that at least 20% of school-aged children have difficulty maintaining age-appropriate academic performance. When a young patient presents with school problems, the primary-care physician should consider difficulties in five potential areas: (1) intelligence, (2) academic achievement, (3) attention/concentration, (4) perceptual (visual–motor) function, and (5) behavioral. Two major contributors to poor academic achievement are learning disabilities (LDs) and mental retardation (MR).

The U.S. Department of Education reported that 4.36 million children in this country received some type of special education service during the 1984–1985 school year.[1] The number of school children identified as learning disabled from 1976 to 1986 increased from 797,000 to 1,925,000.[2] It is estimated that the yearly increase in learning-disabled children exceeds that for all other handicapping conditions combined. Surprisingly, many learning-disability placements occur between the ages of 6 and 11, but more than twice as many occur after age 11. The Centers for Disease Control estimate that the prevalence of learning disabilities is approximately 5% to 10% of the school-aged population[3] (mental retardation occurs in 2–3% of this population).

Learning-disabled children, as a group, represent almost 50% of all children served under Public Law 94-142, the Education for All Handicapped Children Act.[4] This law was intended to be an educational "bill of rights" for handicapped children, providing for an appropriate education. The law originally encompassed children 5 to 18 years of age and required identification, diagnosis, and provision of educational and related services. The age range was extended from 3 to 21 years in 1977, although services for children between 3 and 5 years remained optional. Handicapping conditions eligible for services under PL 94-142 include mental retardation, hearing deficits, speech and language disorders, specific learning disabilities, visual handicaps, emotional disturbance, orthopedic problems, and "other health-impaired" medical conditions.

Under PL 94-142, each child is evaluated by a multidisciplinary team, with an Individual Education Plan (IEP) being formulated (to be reviewed annually). The child must be placed in the "least restrictive" environment ("mainstreamed" as much as possible), and related services must be provided (transportation, physical therapy, occupational therapy, speech pathology). Parents and children have rights to "due process" in case of disagreement in regard to programming. A reevaluation must be repeated every 3 years.[5]

Public Law 99-457, the Education of the Handicapped Act Amendments of 1986,[6] further extended the range of this law by mandating that services be provided for children 3 to 5 years of age. States were offered the option to serve children with handicaps or developmental delays from birth to 3 years of age. This law was more family centered than PL 94-142 (which primarily focuses on the child), and an Individualized Family Service Plan (IFSP) was devised.[7]

As indicated in Chapter 2, Public Law 99-457 was replaced with the Individuals with Disabilities Act of 1990 (IDEA; PL 101-476). In addition to mandating that intervention services be provided for young children, "transition services" also were mandated for students in special education who are 16 years of age or older. Provision of transition services is defined as a process that promotes movement from school to postschool activities (e.g., postsecondary education, vocational training, employment, or independent living).[8]

6.2. DEFINING LEARNING DISABILITIES

Despite federal regulations, the definition of "LDs" still is controversial. According to PL 94-142, a specific learning disability

> . . . means a disorder in one or more of the basic psychological processes involved in the understanding or in using language, spoken or written, which may manifest itself in an imperfect ability to listen, think, speak, read, write, spell, or to do mathematical calculations. The term includes such conditions as perceptual handicaps, brain injury, minimal brain dysfunction, dyslexia, and developmental aphasia. The term does not apply to children who have learning problems

which are primarily the result of visual, hearing, or motor handicaps, of mental retardation, or emotional disturbance, or of environmental, cultural, or economic disadvantages.[4]

Public Law 94-142 stipulated that the child must have a severe *discrepancy* between intellectual ability and academic achievement in order to be classified as learning disabled. This regulation has become a major identification criterion for establishing LD eligibility. In many states, the quantification of this discrepancy has become quite elaborate; between 1981 and 1985, the increased reliance on aptitude/achievement formulas generated the need for more stringent discrepancy criteria.[9] This, in part, reflected the necessity to limit the number of learning-disabled students identified and placed in special programs, thereby decreasing educational costs.

Defining LDs, as noted, is a highly controversial topic. The issue initially surfaced in 1962 with Kirk's[10] first effort to delineate the term "learning disability." The definition can be either conceptual or operational; regardless, it is significant because it focuses advocacy efforts and ensures provision of services. Learning disabilities may be viewed from different perspectives by various disciplines; this results in an inability to formulate a definition that is universally acceptable.

A review of 28 recent editions of textbooks that deal with learning disabilities revealed 11 different, but frequently used, definitions.[11] Although all definitions emphasize that the child with a learning disability is an underachiever, each varies on other important issues such as central nervous system dysfunction, etiology, process involvement, and specification of LDs as verbal language problems, academic problems, or conceptual problems.[11] The definition formulated by the National Joint Committee on Learning Disabilities[12] is probably the best available at this time and the one with the best possibility of becoming the "consensus definition"[11]:

> Learning disabilities is a general term that refers to a heterogeneous group of disorders manifested by significant difficulties in the acquisition and use of listening, speaking, reading, writing, reasoning, or mathematical abilities. These disorders are intrinsic to the individual, presumed to be due to central nervous system dysfunction, and may occur across the life span. Problems in self-regulatory behaviors, social perception, and social interaction may exist with learning disabilities but do not by themselves constitute a learning disability. Although learning disabilities may occur concomitantly with other handicapping conditions (for example, sensory impairment, mental retardation, serious emotional disturbance) or with extrinsic influences (such as cultural differences, insufficient or inappropriate instruction), they are not the result of those conditions or influences.[12] (p. 1)

Of note is the fact that the psychiatric definition of learning disability (one that primary-care physicians will encounter and that is necessary for completion of medical and insurance forms) differs markedly from both federal and state classification systems.[13] Rather than focus on the underlying learning problems, DSM-III-R[14] emphasizes the areas of academic difficulty, namely, the Specific Developmental Disorders. Subgroupings of these disorders include (1) Academic Skills Disorders (developmental arithmetic, expressive writing, reading disorder), (2) Language and Speech Disorders (developmental articulation, expressive language, receptive language disorder), and (3) Motor Skills Disorder (developmental coordination disorder). The DSM-III-R accepts that one could have mental retardation *and* learning disabilities as coexisting problems, a concept that is not accepted in the federal regulations. Unfortunately, the use of the DSM-III-R criteria may cause interpretive problems when "conversing" with school systems.

It appears that learning disabilities are heterogeneous problems, probably caused by subtle central nervous system processing dysfunctions, and may occur in conjunction with secondary sequelae. Learning disability is an educational rather than a medical diagnosis. Whether or not LDs can occur in association with compromised intellectual function continues to be a debatable issue.

6.3. THE DISCREPANCY ISSUE

Primary-care physicians should become familiar with the "discrepancy issue," as this has been established as the primary criterion for identifying children with learning disabilities. Frequently parents will request advice and interpretation of this concept. Unfortunately, discrepancy formulas are controversial, potentially inaccurate, and inappropriate for detecting cognitive deficits.[15] Essentially, there are three types of discrepancies: aptitude–achievement, intracognitive, and intra-achievement.[16]

6.3.1. Aptitude–Achievement Discrepancy

An aptitude–achievement discrepancy reflects the disparity between a child's intellectual ability and actual level of academic achievement. Generally, IQ scores are compared to levels of academic achievement, which are derived from standardized tests (see Chapter 8 regarding achievement testing).

For example, if a child's intelligence quotient were 100 (average) and the standard score (see Chapter 1) in reading obtained on a measure of academic achievement were 70 (approximately 2 SD below average), the difference or discrepancy between these two estimates would be significant. Generally, based on the IQ estimate, one would expect the reading and IQ scores to be comparable, and therefore, both to fall in the average range. In this case, the difference between scores is suggestive of a specific dysfunction in reading.

6.3.2. Intracognitive Discrepancy

An intracognitive discrepancy, also called a disturbance in basic "psychological processes," occurs in children who have a *specific* type of cognitive dysfunction such as a deficit in auditory processing, short-term memory, or visual processing. The effects might be limited or general; for example, in the latter scenario an auditory sequential-processing dysfunction might affect auditory short-term memory, reading, and spelling (particularly phonics). Unfortunately, these particular cognitive dysfunctions are difficult to operationalize.

An example of an intracognitive discrepancy is found in a student who experiences difficulty retaining information that is presented verbally by the teacher but who can adequately recall information that is presented visually (i.e., written on the board or demonstrated). Although many children have a preference for a specific mode of instruction, the existence of an *inability* to perform adequately in one area in contrast to appropriate skills in other areas is indicative of an intracognitive discrepancy.

6.3.3. Intra-Achievement Discrepancy

An intra-achievement discrepancy reflects divergence or inconsistency in educational achievement performances. This type of discrepancy could occur between academic areas (e.g., reading is significantly higher or lower than mathematics skills) or within an academic area (such as a marked difference between reading decoding and reading comprehension).

Therefore, a child whose standard scores or grade equivalents in reading decoding and spelling are lower than those for reading comprehension demonstrates an intra-achievement discrepancy. Similarly, it is not unusual for the clinician to encounter a child whose achievement level in mathematics is lower than those in all other areas. Again, this circumscribed deficit is indicative of an intra-achievement discrepancy.

6.3.4. Specific Issues

There are specific issues concerning the "discrepancy concept" that are noteworthy. In the aptitude–achievement discrepancy, learning disabilities may also affect a child's performance on IQ tests, thereby reducing the discrepancy between aptitude and achievement. In particular, this would be the case in the presence of a short-term memory or central-processing dysfunction and in the most severe LDs. Unfortunately, failure to demonstrate a significant "discrepancy" (even though one exists) would preclude eligibility for services.

Retrieval memory dysfunction, organizational or attention problems, or fine motor dyspraxia usually are not detected with discrepancy formulas.[17] Moreover, aptitude–achievement and intracognitive discrepancies have increased significance in the identification of learning-disabled children from grade 3 onwards.[15] Children, by this grade level and above, fall further and further below their estimated ability and would be more likely to reveal a discrepancy. However, an intracognitive discrepancy is most useful in the identification of preschool and primary-age children who have learning disabilities. Generally, use of the aptitude–achievement discrepancy often precludes early intervention.[15] Moreover, the discrepancy criteria do not provide clinicians with the opportunity to discriminate among the various problems that children encounter in learning.

The aptitude–achievement discrepancy, despite widespread use, probably should not form the primary criterion for determining a learning disability. Definitions must incorporate consideration of intracognitive dysfunctions as well. Viewing learning disabilities as a general, heterogeneous category and then identifying the specific type of dysfunction (analogous to identifying an illness as viral and then further defining it as rubella, mumps, or varicella) are most appropriate.[15] An aptitude–achievement discrepancy may be considered a sufficient criterion for LD but not a necessary one.

Regression models, which attempt to correct the problems inherent in discrepancy models, are now used in 13 of the 30 states that have set specific criteria for determining a severe discrepancy. In regression equations, the statistical relationship between IQ and achievement is considered. In general, there is a decreased probability of a simple discrepancy when a child's IQ is low; there is a greater likelihood of a discrepancy when the student's IQ is high. With the regression model, there is an equal probability that a discrepancy will be identified across IQ levels. Given that the majority of referrals for poor school achievement involve children with lower IQs, use of simple discrepancy models results in underidentification of children with learning disabilities; use of regression equations may increase the identification rate by as much as 10%.

Primary-care physicians also should be aware that grade equivalents, often used in the determination of learning disabilities, are controversial (Chapter 1). This controversy occurs because of misinterpretation of these derived scores and the lack of appropriate statistical properties. Although grade equivalents routinely are used because of their appeal for potential demonstration of positive gains, it has been shown that teachers and school psychologists are less likely to classify hypothetical cases as learning disabled when grade equivalents, versus percentiles or standard scores, are used.[18,19] Interpretation of grade equivalents is particularly problematic past seventh or eighth grade.[20] It is recommended that practitioners use grade equivalents in conjunction with standard scores and percentiles whenever interpretation of academic achievement is necessary.

6.4. ANCILLARY LD ISSUES

Primary-care physicians who work with children with learning disabilities also must address associated family issues. An awareness of the various psychostressors that potentially may be problematic is necessary. Results of interviews with parents of LD children have enumerated several major areas of concern,[21] including (1) how the parent(s) might be involved in the child's education, (2) parent–school relationships, (3) need for external supports (from family, friends, and professional organizations), (4) emotional strains of parenting the child with learning disabilities, and (5) social concerns about the LD child (e.g., his/her embarrassment about the disability and need for special education).

Parents, as a rule, have numerous questions related to the later outcome of LD children who have received special educational help.[22] It has been estimated that 250,000 to 300,000 students with LDs graduate from school each year; 30% of students enrolled in secondary special-education programs drop out of school.[23] There appears to be a major shortcoming in the availability of postsecondary services. Those LD students who are being graduated are rarely eligible for programs that provide service for disabled adults. Unfortunately, the need for special services does not terminate on graduation from high school. In a recent study of 64 LD graduates (mean age 21 years), the majority (79%) were living at home or with relatives; 9% were married and living with a spouse; and approximately 70% possessed a driver's license. However, 31% were unemployed.[22] Most of the LD graduates who were working were not employed full time, and salaries generally were low. Few had a wide range of leisure pursuits and/or social contacts.[22]

These inadequacies in employment, residential environment, and psychosocial growth were probably not the result of deficiencies in public school education programs but, rather, reflect the negative effects of the paucity of comprehensive community services. Parental attitudes about their learning-disabled child's independence and competitive employment also are critical. Parents must be advised not to be overly restrictive or protective.

6.5. MENTAL RETARDATION

Mental retardation (MR), as well as learning disabilities, are components in the spectrum of developmental disabilities that may negatively affect educational achievement. Since mental retardation occurs in 2% to 3% of the general population and is diagnosed in more than 780,000 school-aged children, the issue warrants discussion. Of particular interest to the primary-care physician is an awareness that 89% of mentally retarded children display mild mental retardation (IQs between 2 and 3 SD below average; 55–69 range). This level of retardation appears to be more strongly related to polygenetic, social, and environmental conditions than to pregnancy or birth events.[24] Causes of severe mental retardation are primarily genetic, biochemical, viral, and developmental (severe mental retardation is not typically related to birth effects). In general, only if there is an association with cerebral palsy is severe retardation linked to asphyxia.[24] Parents will often question the physician regarding the etiology of the retardation; unfortunately, in the majority of cases the etiology cannot be determined.

In educational classifications, mild mental retardation (IQ 55–69) is termed "educable," moderate mental retardation (IQ in the 40–54 range; 6% of MR population) is termed "trainable," and severe and profound mental retardation (IQ ≤39; 5% of MR population) is classified as "custodial." It is estimated that educable mentally retarded children will plateau at a sixth-grade educational level, whereas trainable MR children may achieve a second- to fourth-grade level of functioning (see Table 6.1). As can be seen in the table, the level of retardation varies, depending on the standard deviation of the intelligence test that is used.

Again, as was indicated in Chapter 4, both the child's level of intelligence and level of adaptive behavior should be considered in the diagnosis of mental retardation. However, this procedure is not endorsed unanimously, because in many cases discrepancies occur between the two

TABLE 6.1. Classification of Mental Retardation

Level of mental retardation	Educational categorization	IQ range	Ceiling mental age/grade level	Percentage of retarded population
Mild	Educable	69–55[a] 67–52[b]	8–3 to 10–9/sixth grade	89%
Moderate	Trainable	54–40[a] 51–36[b]	5–7 to 8–2/second to fourth grade	6%
Severe	Trainable/custodial	39–25[a] 35–20[b]	3–2 to 5–6/no functional academic skills	3.5%
Profound	Custodial	<25[a] <20[b]	<3–2/needs total care	1.5%

[a]IQ on WISC-III, WISC-R, or WPPSI (SD = 15).
[b]IQ on Stanford–Binet IV (SD = 16).

domains. Generally, the assessment of intelligence and resultant IQ scores are more reliable and valid than are data obtained in the evaluation of adaptive behavior. Nonetheless, use of both criteria decreases the number of children diagnosed as mentally retarded in comparison to numbers of children diagnosed by use of IQ estimates only.

In the past, it was believed that although children with mental retardation display a slower rate and a compromised ultimate level of development, their overall cognitive growth pattern is similar to that found in children without retardation.[25] However, more recent evidence suggests that developmental rates vary among mentally retarded children from different etiological groups.[26] For example, children with Down syndrome exhibit a progressive decrease in their rate of development that begins during infancy. This decline is most evident in language function. In contrast, males with fragile X syndrome experience a slowing of cognitive development between 10 and 15 years of age.[26] Therefore, the practitioner should not view the population of children with mental retardation as being homogeneous.

Practitioners should be aware that one of the largest groups of children with problems in academic performance are those who are categorized as "slow learners." These students are sometimes classified as having "borderline intelligence," typically with IQs between one and two standard deviations below average (IQ 70–85 range). These children, who are not classified as mentally retarded, tend to remain in regular classrooms. It is not assured that they will receive special education assistance because they do not meet federal eligibility criteria. Frequently, these children are required to repeat grades, and they are expected to exhibit a slow rate of learning. Children who fit into the "slow learner" range often are classified as "learning disabled" so as to receive services (although they are not truly LD). Unfortunately, a significant number of these children simply "fall through the cracks" and experience continued frustrations during their school years.

A clue that mental retardation is the etiological origin for poor school performance resides in comparably low IQ, levels of academic achievement, visual–motor integrative skills, and adaptive functioning (see Chapter 4). Crocker and Nelson[27] provide a meaningful discussion of MR in behavioral pediatrics. Physicians generally are sensitive to the connotations of the term "mentally retarded" and the fact that it is viewed as stigmatizing by many parents. Therefore, many practitioners are reluctant to use the term. Special precautions must be taken not to categorically and erroneously apply this term to minority children and/or children from depressed socioeconomic environments. "Developmental delay" is a term that is often used even in characterizing older children with mental retardation.[28]

6.6. SUMMARY

It has been estimated that the number of young Americans with chronic physical conditions include: chronic bronchitis, 3.5 million; asthma, 3.2 million; orthopedic impairments, 1.8 million, and heart murmurs, 1.1 million.[28] According to the most recent estimates derived from the National Health Interview Survey of Child Health (NHIS-CH),[28] 2.5 million children have developmental delays (4% of children aged 17 years and younger), and 3.4 million have a learning disability (6.5% of children of the same age). A total of 19.5% of children ages 3 to 17 years (nearly 10.2 million) have one or more developmental, learning, or emotional disorders. Moreover, 35% of children ages 3 to 17 years who were described by their parents as exhibiting "fair or poor health" had developmental, learning, or behavioral problems.[28] The high prevalence of these disorders appears to be increasing. These disorders are significant challenges for health care professionals, since they are not transient and/or inconsequential; they affect the child, family, and society.

The two major disorders associated with problems in school performance, namely learning disabilities and mental retardation, also display different age trends. In the NHIS-CH study, the median age at which delays in development were first noted was 14 months; 45% of delays were detected before the child's first birthday. In contrast, the median age at which learning disabilities were first recognized was 6 years 7 months;

45% were first noted between the ages of 6 and 8 years.[28] However, in 16% of the children with learning disabilities, the LDs were not detected until late elementary or secondary school. Although mental retardation occurs somewhat more frequently in males than in females, the sex difference is not great (4.2% of males versus 3.8% of females). On the other hand, LDs are twice as frequent in males than in females (8.6% versus 4.4%).[28]

There appears to be an increased prevalence of learning disabilities over the last decade. Possible reasons for this increase have been debated, particularly in light of a corresponding decrease in the identification of mental retardation and speech or language impairments.[29,30] It is possible that the relative "newness" of the learning-disabilities discipline has had some influence.[31] More specifically, professionals have become more adept at recognizing children with learning disabilities. Social/cultural changes also have been implicated as a cause for the increased prevalence of LDs.[31] It is speculated that social/cultural changes may have (1) placed the children's central nervous systems at increased risk for disruption and (2) placed an increased degree of psychosocial stress on children and their families, thereby negatively affecting the children's social support networks.[31] Hallahan recently characterized learning disabilities as "one of the most sensitive barometers of the biomedical status of children and the psychosocial climate in which they live"[31] (p. 524). Pediatricians also must consider that some of the increase in prevalence of LDs may result from misdiagnosis; however, there is ample evidence to suggest that some of this increase is real.

In the following chapters, descriptions are provided of assessment instruments frequently used in the evaluation of problems in school performance. These test instruments are grouped into five general assessment areas: (1) intelligence (Chapter 7), (2) academic achievement (Chapter 8), (3) attention/concentration (Chapter 9), (4) perceptual function (Chapter 10), and (5) behavioral (Chapter 11).

REFERENCES

1. U.S. Department of Education, 1986, *Eighth Annual Report to Congress on the Implementation of Public Law 94-142: The Education for All Handicapped Children Act*, U.S. Department of Education, Washington, DC.
2. U.S. Department of Education, 1987, *Ninth Annual Report to Congress on the Implementation of the Education of the Handicapped Act*, U.S. Department of Education, Washington, DC.
3. Interagency Committee on Learning Disabilities, 1987, *Learning Disabilities: A Report to the U.S. Congress*, Department of Health and Human Services, Washington, DC.
4. U.S. Congress, 1977, The Education for All Handicapped Children Act of 1975, PL 94-142; 20 U.S.C. 1401, et seq., *Fed. Register* **42**:42474–42518.

5. Committee on Children with Disabilities, 1987, Pediatrician's role in development and implementation of an individual education plan, *Pediatrics* **80:**750–751.

6. Education of the Handicapped Act Amendments, 1986, *Report to Accompany H.R. 5520, Report 98-860,* U.S. House of Representatives, Washington, DC.

7. DeGraw, C., Edell, D., Ellers, B., Hillemeier, M., Liebman, J., et al., 1988, Public Law 99-457: New opportunities to serve young children with special needs, *J. Pediatr.* **113:** 971–974.

8. Destefano, L., 1992, IDEA. Assessment for transition, *Child Assess. News* **2:**1–10.

9. Frankenberger, W., and Harper, J., 1987, States' criteria and procedures for identifying learning disabled children: A comparison of 1981/82 and 1985/86 guidelines, *J. Learn. Dis.* **20:**118–121.

10. Kirk, S. A., and Bateman, B., 1962, Diagnosis and remediation of learning disabilities, *Except. Child* **29:**73–78.

11. Hammill, D. D., 1990, On defining learning disabilities: An emerging consensus, *J. Learn. Dis.* **23:**74–91.

12. National Joint Committee on Learning Disabilities, 1988, Letter to NJCLD member organizations, p. 1.

13. Silver, L. B., 1989, Learning disabilities, *J. Am. Acad. Child Adol. Psychiat.* **28:**309–313.

14. American Psychiatric Association, 1987, *Diagnostic and Statistical Manual of Mental Disorders,* ed. 3, revised, American Psychiatric Association, Washington, DC.

15. Mather, N., and Healey, W. C., 1989, Deposing aptitude-achievement discrepancy as the imperial criterion for learning disabilities, *Learn. Dis.* **1:**40–48.

16. Woodcock, R. W., 1984, A response to some questions raised about the Woodcock–Johnson, *School Psychol. Rev.* **13:**355–362.

17. Levine, M. D., 1989, Learning disabilities at 25: The early adulthood of a maturing concept, *Learn. Dis.* **1:**1–11.

18. Huebner, S., 1988, Bias in teachers' special education decisions as a function of test score reporting format, *J. Ed. Res.* **81:**217–220.

19. Huebner, S., 1989, Errors in decision making: A comparison of school psychologists' interpretations of grade equivalents, percentiles, and deviation IQs, *School Psychol. Rev.* **18:**51–55.

20. Green, D. R., 1987, Interpreting test scores from standardized achievement tests, *Natl. Assoc. Second. School Bull.* **71:**23–35.

21. Waggoner, L., and Wilgosh, L., 1990, Concerns of families of children with learning disabilities, *J. Learn. Dis.* **23:**97–113.

22. Haring, K. A., Lovett, D. L., and Smith, D. D., 1990, A follow-up study of recent special education graduates of learning disabilities programs, *J. Learn. Dis.* **23:**108–112.

23. Will, M., 1984, *OSERS Programming for the Transition of Youth with Disabilities: Bridges from School to Working Life,* Office of Special Education and Rehabilitative Services, U.S. Department of Education, Washington, DC.

24. Task Force on Joint Assessment of Prenatal and Perinatal Factors Associated with Brain Disorders, 1985 statement, National Institutes of Health report on causes of mental retardation and cerebral palsy, *Pediatrics* **76:**457–458.

25. Zigler, E., 1969, Developmental versus different theories of mental retardation and the problem of motivation, *Am. J. Ment. Defic.* **73:**536–566.

26. Bregman, J. D., and Hodapp, R. M., 1991, Current developments in the understanding of mental retardation. Part I: Biological and phenomenological perspectives, *J. Am. Acad. Child. Adol. Psychiat.* **30:**707–719.

27. Crocker, A. C., and Nelson, R. P., 1983, Mental retardation, in: *Developmental–Behavioral*

Pediatrics (M. L. Levine, W. B. Carey, A. C. Crocker, and R. T. Gross, eds.), W. B. Saunders, New York, pp. 756–770.

28. Zill, N., and Schoenborn, C. A., 1990, *Developmental, Learning, and Emotional Problems. Health of Our Nation's Children, United States, 1988, Advance Data from Vital and Health Statistics: No. 190*, National Center for Health Statistics, Hyattsville, MD.

29. U.S. Department of Education, 1990, *Twelfth Annual Report to Congress on the Implementation of the Education of the Handicapped Act*, U.S. Department of Education, Washington, DC.

30. U.S. Department of Education, 1991, *Thirteenth Annual Report to Congress on the Implementation of the Individuals with Disabilities Education Act*, U.S. Department of Education, Washington, DC.

31. Hallahan, D. P., 1992, Some thoughts on why the prevalence of learning disabilities has increased, *J. Learn. Dis.* **25:**523–528.

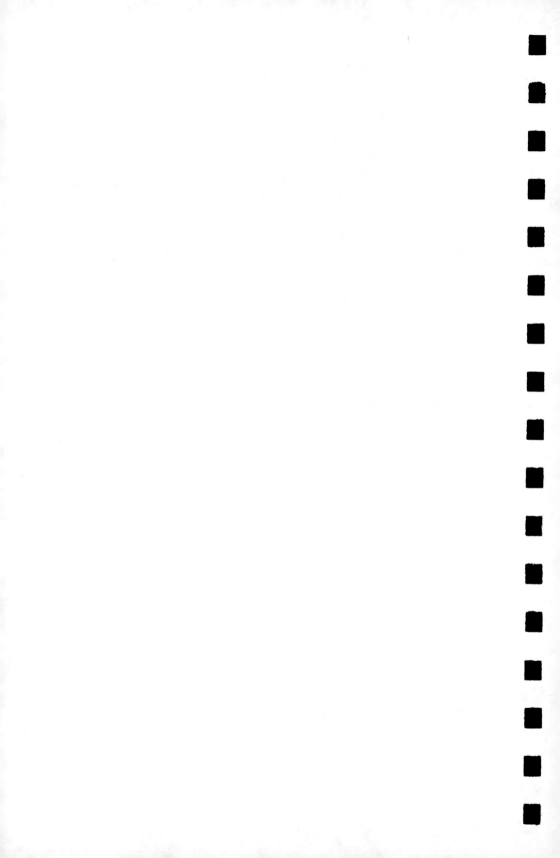

7 ❃ Assessment of Cognitive/Intellectual Functioning

7.1. INTRODUCTION

A wide variety of psychological test instruments exist that are used to evaluate intellectual functioning. The description of instruments that follows is not all inclusive; rather, it focuses on tests that are used most frequently in clinical practice and that the primary-care physician will most likely come in contact with (see Table 7.1).

7.2. WECHSLER PRESCHOOL AND PRIMARY SCALE OF INTELLIGENCE-REVISED

The original Wechsler Preschool and Primary Scale of Intelligence[1] (WPPSI), published in 1967, was applicable for ages 4 to 6½ years. Intelligence was viewed as global and multidimensional, and therefore a Verbal IQ (VIQ), Performance IQ (PIQ), and Full-Scale IQ (FSIQ) were provided. The original test was criticized because of its limited "floor", i.e., it did not allow clear differentiation of abilities at the lower end of the scale (e.g., the lowest IQ that could be obtained at age 4 was 55).[2]

The WPPSI was replaced in 1989 by the WPPSI-R,[1] which retained 48% of the original test items. The age range of the WPPSI-R was extended to include children ages 3 years to 7 years 3 months (see Figure 7.1). The upper age range of the WPPSI-R overlaps (by 1 year) the lower age range of the Wechsler Intelligence Scale for Children—Revised (WISC-R) and the Wechsler Intelligence Scale—Third Edition (to be reviewed later in this chapter). It is recommended that if there is a question whether the child is below average in intelligence or communicative skills, the WPPSI-R should

TABLE 7.1. Tests of Cognitive/Intellectual Functioning

Test	Year	Ages	Publisher	Administration
Wechsler Preschool and Primary Scale of Intelligence-Revised (WPPSI-R)	1989	3 yr to 7 yr 3 mo	The Psychological Corporation, San Antonio, TX	Psychologist
Wechsler Intelligence Scale for Children-Revised (WISC-R)	1974	6 yr to 16 yr 11 mo	The Psychological Corporation, San Antonio, TX	Psychologist
Wechsler Intelligence Scale for Children-Third Edition (WISC-III)	1991	6 yr to 16 yr 11 mo	The Psychological Corporation, San Antonio, TX	Psychologist
Stanford–Binet-Fourth Edition (SB-4)	1986	2 yr to adult	Riverside Publishing, Chicago, IL	Psychologist
Kaufman Assessment Battery for Children (K-ABC)	1983	2½ to 12½ yr	American Guidance Service, Circle Pines, MN	Psychologist
Wide-Range Assessment of Memory and Learning	1990	5 to 17 yr	Jastek Associates, Wilmington, DE	Psychologist/ other professionals
Kaufman Brief Intelligence Test (K-BIT)	1990	4 to 9 yr	American Guidance Service, Circle Pines, MN	Various professionals

be the test instrument of choice in this overlapping 6- to 7-year age range; otherwise, the WISC-R or WISC-III would be the preferred test.[3,4] At the lower end, the WPPSI-R overlaps the Bayley Scales of Infant Development II (which is applicable up to 42 months of age).

The WPPSI-R was normed on a stratified sample of 2100 children. It contains 12 subtests (two are optional), divided into performance and verbal scales. Therefore, a PIQ, VIQ, and FSIQ are obtained (M = 100, SD = 15); the mean subtest scaled score is 10 (SD = 3). WPPSI-R IQ scores range from 41 to 160; ≥120 is considered superior, 110 to 119 high average, 90 to 109 average, and 80 to 89 low average. Essentially the same tests are administered at each age, although specific tasks and scoring criteria vary. This test requires 75 to 90 min to administer.

7.2.1. Performance Subtests[1,3,5]

- *Object Assembly*. The examinee is required to fit pieces of puzzles together (e.g., automobile). This subtest, which contains six full-

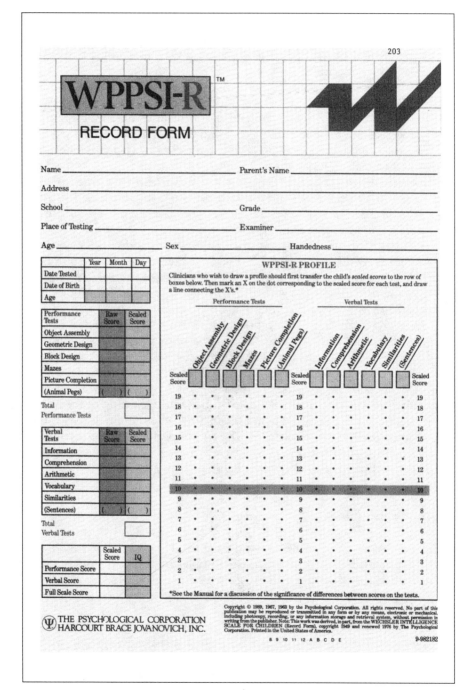

FIGURE 7.1. Face sheet from the Wechsler Preschool and Primary Scale of Intelligence. (Copyright 1989, 1967, 1963 by the Psychological Corporation. Reproduced by permission. All rights reserved.)

color puzzles of common objects, evaluates eye–hand coordination, perceptual organization, and the ability to assemble parts of a concrete object into a whole.

- *Geometric Design*. This test contains two parts: (1) visual recognition/discrimination and (2) copying figures. In the former, the child looks at a design and selects a similar one from an array of four designs. In the second part, the child is required to reproduce designs from a printed model (e.g., square). Visual perception, visual–motor integrative skills, and attention to detail are assessed.
- *Block Design*. The main requirement of this task is to arrange and reproduce geometric patterns with flat two-colored blocks. Psychomotor speed, visual–spatial perception, and synthesis of part–whole information are evaluated.
- *Mazes*. The youngster is presented with paper-and-pencil mazes of increasing difficulty. The child's score is determined by the number of errors made; however, the floor of the Mazes subtest is weak for younger children (3-year-olds). This subtest measures fine motor skills, visual planning, and visual perceptual abilities.
- *Picture Completion*. Pictures of common objects are presented in which details are missing. This task assesses the child's ability to recognize what part is missing from these pictures (face without a nose, clock without hands). Primary skills that are measured include attention to detail, visual organization, and long-term visual memory.
- *Animal Pegs*. This optional test requires rapid learning of the association between colored pegs and pictures of four animals, based on a key (e.g., cat = black peg). The child's performance is scored in terms of speed and accuracy. This task measures memory, attention, concentration, and fine motor coordination.

7.2.2. Verbal Subtests[1,3–5]

- *Information*. This subtest measures general knowledge of events or objects in the environment. For example, the child is requested to give names of several fruits, days of week, or body parts. In addition to general knowledge, this subtest measures verbal fluency and long-term memory.
- *Comprehension*. The child is asked to provide verbal expressions of reasons for activities, actions, or consequences of events (e.g., Why shouldn't you touch a hot object? Why do we need to bathe?). Verbal ability and logical reasoning are involved.
- *Arithmetic*. This test requires demonstration of an understanding of

basic quantitative concepts from simple counting to solving word problems (e.g., counting eight blocks, answering questions such as: If you had three balloons and one of them broke, how many would you have left?). Knowledge of numerical concepts is involved.

- *Vocabulary*. This subtest contains two parts: (1) naming or identifying pictures and (2) defining words. Words such as tree, coat, and book are included in the latter part. Verbal fluency and formal education are influential on this subtest.

- *Similarities*. On the similarities subtest, the concept of "sameness" is measured in an increasingly abstract fashion. In the first section, a picture is selected that is most similar to a group of pictured objects that share common features. In the second section, the child must complete a verbally presented sentence that reflects a similarity between two things. In the third section, the child must verbally describe how two things are similar (e.g., peach and plum). Visual organization, logical reasoning, verbal fluency, and concept formation are involved.

- *Sentences*. This optional test measures short-term auditory memory by having the student repeat verbatim a sentence read by the examiner. Verbal facility and memory are involved.

Physicians reviewing WPPSI-R test data should be aware that 95% confidence limits for the PIQ is ±9 points, VIQ ±7 points, and FSIQ ±6 points. An 11-point VIQ/PIQ discrepancy,[6] however, is not atypical. It is recommended that a minimum of 6 months must elapse before WPPSI-R retesting: 1 year is preferred.[6] Although the WPPSI-R is highly correlated with the original WPPSI ($r = 0.87$), children tend to score lower on the WPPSI-R. This discrepancy is 8 points on the FSIQ, 9 points on the PIQ, and 5 points on the VIQ.[3] Children will score lower on the WPPSI-R than on the WISC-R despite a good correlation between the two test instruments ($r = 0.85$). The WPPSI-R is significantly correlated with the McCarthy Scales ($r = 0.81$) and other tests of preschool intelligence.[1,3,4]

In summary, there are several weaknesses in regard to the WPPSI-R: (1) it requires a relatively long administration time (60 min), and (2) the lowest IQ score of 41 is not possible to obtain below age 5 years and 8 months even if the child does not give any correct answers.[7] On the positive side, the test extends the Wechsler series from 3 years to 75 years (adult version). In addition, the downward extension is useful for the PL 99-457 mandate, which has resulted in an increased number of preschoolers being referred for early assessment. The WPPSI-R generally is viewed as a good preschool test by psychometricians, perhaps even the "test of choice"[8] for evaluation in this age range.

7.3. WECHSLER INTELLIGENCE SCALE FOR CHILDREN-REVISED

The IQ test most frequently administered to school-aged children has been the Wechsler Intelligence Scale for Children-Revised[9] (WISC-R). The original WISC, first published in 1949, and the WISC-R[9] (instituted in 1974) have had more than 1100 articles published concerning them. The age range for administration of the WISC-R is 6 years through 16 years 11 months. As in the case of the WPPSI-R, the WISC-R provides a Verbal, Performance, and Full-Scale IQ (M = 100, SD = 15). These also are deviation IQs, obtained by comparing the examinee's scores to those obtained by a representative sample of same-aged peers. The IQ scores range from 40 to 160; scores 130 and above are considered very superior, those 120 to 129 superior, 110 to 119 high average, 90 to 109 average, 80 to 89 low average, 70 to 79 borderline, and 69 cognitively deficient.[9] The WISC-R overlaps with the Wechsler Adult Intelligence Scale (WAIS-R)[10] in the 16-year to 16-year 11-month age range. It is recommended that the WISC-R be used in lieu of the WAIS-R with adolescents who are suspected of having below-average intelligence because it allows for a more thorough sampling of abilities.[2]

The WISC-R was normed on a stratified sample of 2200 children. Like the WPPSI, it contains 12 subtests, six verbal and six performance. Scaled scores have a M of 10 and SD of 3. The same tests are administered at each age, although specific tasks and scoring criteria will vary. Administration time is approximately 60 min, depending on age and level of functioning.

7.3.1. Verbal Subtests[2,9]

- *Information*. The information subtest contains 30 items that measure a child's fund of general information. Factual questions include items such as: In which direction does the sun rise? On what continent is Brazil? How many nickels make a quarter?
- *Similarities*. This task consists of 17 items that measure abstract concept-formation skills. The child is requested to describe in what way a foot and a yard are alike, a magazine and a book, or a dog and a cat.
- *Arithmetic*. Ability to perform "mental" arithmetic computations is measured on this subtest. The last three of the 18 tasks require that the child read and solve word problems (e.g., at 25 cents per pack, how much will six packs of gum cost?).

- *Vocabulary*. Vocabulary and verbal fluency skills are assessed on this subtest. It is the best measure of overall intelligence of the verbal tasks. The child is requested to define various words from a series of 32 words presented by the examiner.
- *Comprehension*. The comprehension subtest contains 17 questions that measure verbal practical reasoning skills. Hypothetical questions involving interpersonal relations, social mores, and factual information are presented (e.g., what should you do if you see a small child by a busy street who is unattended?).
- *Digit Span*. This optional test measures attention and short-term auditory memory; the child is required to repeat series of digits (ranging from three to nine) forwards and to repeat series in a reverse fashion (ranging in length from two to eight). The latter task also measures dual conceptual tracking. Although an optional subtest, it is recommended that this test be administered routinely.

7.3.2. Performance Subtests

- *Picture Completion*. This subtest measures the child's ability to detect environmental nuances visually. Twenty-six drawings of objects or persons are presented, and the requirement is to indicate the missing part (e.g., picture of a truck without a tire, a face without a mouth).
- *Picture Arrangement*. The subtest measures nonverbal practical reasoning skills. The task utilizes 12 short "comic strip" series that are presented under timed conditions. The child must place pictures (ranging from three to five) in the correct sequence to depict a story (e.g., a person getting dressed).
- *Block Design*. On this task, two-dimensional red and white blocks must be placed into designated designs (copied) within time limits. The 11 items comprising this subtest measure nonverbal abstract concept formation skills as well as visual–perceptual abilities. Block design is the best measure of general intelligence of all performance subtests on the WISC-R.
- *Object Assembly*. This timed task requires the assembly of four jigsaw puzzles and measures the child's ability to assemble parts of a concrete object into a whole (e.g., boy, truck, animal).
- *Coding*. This test requires the copying of signs and symbols, utilizing a paper-and-pencil format. For children younger than 8 years, shapes and symbols are paired in a key, with the child being allowed 2 min to fill in as many pairs as possible (e.g., a circle contains two

vertical lines, a square has one horizontal line). Older children are required to pair numerals and symbols. This task incorporates a learning component and involves sustained attention and visual motor integration.
- *Mazes.* This is a supplementary test that involves drawing a path out of increasingly complex mazes. The subtest measures both visual planning and visual–motor integrative skills.

A screening version of the WISC-R has been developed[11] that contains two verbal (arithmetic and vocabulary) and two performance subtests (picture arrangement and block design). When subject to factor analysis,[12] WISC-R subtests can be grouped into three factors: (1) verbal comprehension (information, similarities, vocabulary, and comprehension), (2) perceptual organization (picture completion, picture arrangement, block design, object assembly, and mazes), and (3) freedom from distractibility (arithmetic, digit span, and coding). These factors are often utilized in the determination of learning disabilities (LDs).

In the diagnosis of LDs, much emphasis has been placed on the discrepancy between verbal and performance IQs. A 12-point verbal/performance discrepancy occurs by chance in five out of 100 cases (i.e., significant at a $p < 0.05$ level); a 15-point discrepancy is found in one out of 100 cases ($p < 0.01$). The mean verbal-IQ/performance-IQ discrepancy is 9.7 points. Therefore, verbal/performance differences are not, as isolated factors, sufficient to determine LDs. Large differences, however, render the Full-Scale IQ (FSIQ) useless in regard to being a summary statistic.[2,12,13] Kaufman[12] suggested several possibilities that should be considered in the event that such discrepancies occur: (1) sensory deficits, (2) differences in verbal and nonverbal intelligence, (3) differences between fluid and crystallized intelligence, (4) psycholinguistic deficiencies, (5) bilingualism, (6) problems in motor coordination, and (7) socioeconomic factors. Bannatyne[14] produced four WISC-R subtest factors that are helpful in the analysis of learning disabilities: (1) conceptual (similarities, vocabulary, and comprehension), (2) spatial (picture completion, block design, and object assembly), (3) sequential (arithmetic, digit span, and coding), and (4) acquired knowledge (information, arithmetic, and vocabulary). For example, in children with learning disabilities in reading, scores on the factors followed the following sequence: spatial > conceptual > sequential. The so-called ACID subtests (*a*rithmetic, *c*oding, *i*nformation, *d*igit span) have also traditionally been associated with LD assessment.[12]

The pediatrician should recall that 90% confidence intervals for the WISC-R VIQ is ±6, PIQ ±8, and FSIQ ±5. If the WISC-R is read-ministered within 3 months, practice effects will increase scores by 4 to 10 points (mean verbal increase = 4 points, mean performance increment = 10, mean full-scale = 7 points). Those IQs from the original WISC are 4 to 8 points higher than those from the WISC-R; WISC-R IQs are typically 6 points higher than the MSCA General Cognitive Index and 5 to 14 points lower than the WAIS-R.[10]

There is a question as to the cultural fairness of the WISC-R inasmuch as the mean IQ for whites is 102, whereas for blacks it is 86. However, if children are grouped by parental occupation, the mean IQ for children in the highest-socioeconomic-status (SES) group is 108, whereas in the lowest SES group it is 87, regardless of ethnic origin. Therefore, it appears that the PIQ is a better indicator of overall intelligence in more disadvantaged populations. Nonetheless, WISC-R IQ scores correlate well with academic achievement (median correlation = 0.56–0.60) and school grades (0.39).[2]

7.4. WECHSLER INTELLIGENCE SCALE FOR CHILDREN-III

The Wechsler Intelligence Scale for Children-III (WISC-III) recently has become available. This instrument basically is an updated WISC-R containing the same format and subtests but with more current normative data, updated test materials, and revised administration rules.[15] The revision is necessary, as it has been estimated that intelligence quotients generally increase 0.3 points per year.[16] The WISC-III was normed on 2200 individuals and is applicable for ages 6 years to 16 years 11 months. As a result, the WISC-III overlaps the WPPSI-R[1] in the 6- to 7-year age range and overlaps the Wechsler Adult Intelligence Scale-R[10] at 16 years. It is recommended that the WISC-III be used over the WAIS-R in lower-functioning 16-year-olds because the WISC-III has a lower test "floor," and it provides a better estimate of abilities for these students (the lowest IQ is 46, versus 49 to 54 on the WAIS-R). Conversely, the WISC-III should be used instead of the WPPSI-R with bright 6- to 7-year-old children[15] (see Figure 7.2).

In addition to the aforementioned changes, the WISC-III includes a new task, Symbol Search. The task has two levels: "A" for children less than 8 years and "B" for those 8 years and older. Each level contains 45 items. In this task the child visually scans two groups of symbols, a target group (one or two symbols) and a search group (three to five symbols). He/she is required to indicate whether or not a target symbol appears in the search group by marking the appropriate "yes" or "no" box. The task is timed (120 sec), with the child having to respond to figural content of the symbols without any mnemonic techniques being utilized. This task may have particular applicability in attention-deficit assessment (see Figure 7.3).

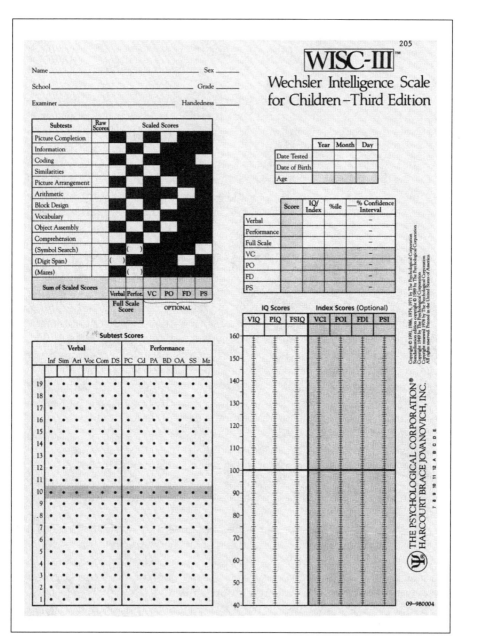

FIGURE 7.2. From the Wechsler Intelligence Scale for Children-Third Edition (WISC-III). (Copyright 1991 by the Psychological Corporation. Reproduced by permission. All rights reserved.)

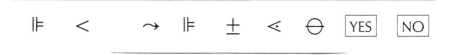

FIGURE 7.3. Sample of the Digit Symbol subtest from the Wechsler Intelligence Scale for Children-Third Edition (WISC-III). (Copyright 1991 by the Psychological Corporation. Reproduced by permission. All rights reserved.)

Factor analysis of the WISC-III has produced four factors[15]: (1) Verbal Comprehension (information, similarities, vocabulary, and comprehension), (2) Perceptual Organization (picture completion, picture arrangement, block design, and object assembly), (3) Freedom from Distractibility (arithmetic and digit span), and (4) Processing Speed (coding and symbol search). A factor score can be obtained for each factor (M = 100, SD = 15), and confidence intervals also are available. This new feature enhances diagnostic accuracy. The mean standard error of measurement for the WISC-III Verbal IQ is 3.53, for the Performance IQ 4.54, and the Full-Scale IQ 3.20.[15] The mean standard errors of measurement for the Verbal Comprehension, Perceptual Organization, Freedom from Distractibility, and Processing Speed Indices are 3.78, 4.68, 5.43, and 5.83 points, respectively.[15]

The WISC-III correlates highly with the WISC-R: $r = 0.90, 0.81$, and 0.89 for the VIQs, PIQs, and FSIQs, respectively. Practitioners can expect the WISC-III FSIQ to be 5 points lower than the WISC-R FSIQ, the VIQ to be 2 points lower, and the PIQ to be 7 points lower than the corresponding WISC-R IQ score. Moreover, differences between scores increase at the upper and lower ends of the IQ distribution. Therefore, a WISC-R FSIQ of 55 would be comparable to a WISC-III IQ of 47 to 54; a WISC-R FSIQ of 70 would correspond to a WISC-III score of 63 to 68, whereas a WISC-R IQ score of 115 would equate to a WISC-III IQ of 108 to 111.[15]

The correlation between the WISC-III and Wechsler Preschool and Primary Scale of Intelligence—Revised (WPPSI-R) is high: $r = 0.85$ for the VIQ and FSIQ, and $r = 0.73$ for the PIQ.[15] However, the WISC-III FSIQ will typically be 4 points greater than the WPPSI-R FSIQ, the VIQ will be 2 points greater, and the PIQ will be 6 points higher.

Correlations between the WISC-III FSIQ scores and group-administered achievement tests such as the Iowa Tests of Basic Skills,[17] the California Achievement Tests,[18] or the Metropolitan Achievement Test[19] are fairly strong ($r = 0.47$).[15] The mean correlation between the WISC-III and school grades is $r = 0.47$.[15]

7.5. STANFORD–BINET-FOURTH EDITION

The original Stanford–Binet Form L-M, first developed in the early 1900s, is the oldest and one of the most frequently used intelligence tests.[2] Until 1960 a ratio IQ was used, i.e., mental age/chronological age × 100. In 1972, updated norms were published that incorporated deviation IQ scores (Chapter 1). The original Stanford–Binet Form L-M, administered from age 2 years through adulthood, yielded a global IQ measure versus definition of areas of specific strengths and weaknesses. As a result, because subtests varied, it was difficult to compare IQs at different ages. For example, the test was heavily loaded with perceptual–performance items in the 3- and 4-year age range, but verbal items were more prevalent at later ages. The Stanford–Binet L-M may continue to serve a limited purpose in the assessment of developmentally delayed toddlers, whose level of function is above the demands of the Bayley Scales but below the basal requirements of the McCarthy Scales.

The Stanford–Binet—Fourth Edition (SB-4),[20-22] normed on more than 5000 subjects, is a revision of the earlier scale. It spans the same age range as the original test, provides basal and ceiling levels, and yields an overall score of general cognitive function. However, the SB-4 differs from the original Stanford–Binet in that there is no age scale, and four area scores are provided in addition to the overall score: (1) verbal reasoning, (2) quantitative reasoning, (3) abstract/visual reasoning, (4) and short-term memory. Theoretically, verbal reasoning and quantitative reasoning are thought to measure crystallized abilities. Abstract/visual reasoning is considered to be a measure of fluid-analytic intelligence.[20,21,23] Short-term memory is felt to be an independent function. The SB-4 contains a total of 15 tests, with the child being administered 8 to 13 of the tests, depending on his/her chronological age. The mean IQ is 100 (SD = 16), and the mean Standard Area Score for each area is 50 (SD = 8). Percentile ranks and age equivalents are also provided. The IQ scores are equated with the following levels of intelligence: ≥132 very superior, 121 to 131 superior, 111 to 120 high average, 89 to 110 average, 79 to 88 low average, 68 to 78 slow learner, and ≤ 67 mentally retarded.[20]

- *Verbal Reasoning Tasks.* There are four verbal reasoning tasks: (1) the 46-item vocabulary subtest (picture vocabulary measuring receptive word knowledge and word definitions that are provided by the child), (2) the 42-item comprehension subtest (identifying body parts, practical problem solving such as understanding basic personal, economic, and social practices), (3) absurdities (selecting inaccurate pictures among three alternatives, verbally explaining what is wrong with the picture), and (4) verbal relations (explanation as to how three words of a four-word set are similar). The verbal relations subtest usually is given to older children (14 years onwards).

- *Quantitative Reasoning*. This area consists of three tasks: (1) quantitative (which contains prearithmetic and arithmetic skills such as counting, addition, subtraction, and other numerical operations), (2) number series (identifying principles underlying series of numbers), and (3) equation building (resequencing numerals and mathematical signs). Equation building is usually administered to children aged 12 years and older.

- *Abstract/Visual Reasoning*. Four subtests are included in this area: (1) pattern analysis (formboards, replication of patterns with blocks), (2) copying (reproduction of block models, copying designs), (3) matrices (a missing matrix figure is indicated from an array), and (4) paper folding/cutting (figures are presented with paper folded and cut; the child chooses among alternatives as to how the paper might look if unfolded). The latter subtest usually is administered to children aged 14 years and older.

- *Short-Term Memory*. This area contains four subtests: (1) bead memory (recall beads that are shown briefly in a photograph, reproduce sequential bead models on a cylindrical rod), (2) memory for sentences (repeat sentences verbatim), (3) memory for digits (recall series of digits forwards and backwards), and (4) memory for objects (pictures of objects are recalled from subsequent displays). The last two tasks typically are administered to children aged 7 years and older.

The SB-4 administration time is 30 to 40 min for preschool-aged children and 60 min for children aged 6 to 11 years. A quick screen version of the SB-4 includes the vocabulary, bead memory, quantitative, and pattern analysis subtests. Median 95% confidence intervals are ±8 for verbal reasoning, ±7 for quantitative reasoning, ±8 for abstract/visual reasoning, ±10 for short-term memory, and ±5 for the composite score.

A major weakness of the SB-4 is the insufficient floor; namely, it is very difficult to identify mild and moderate retardation before the ages of 4 and 5, respectively.[24,25] The original SB could provide this diagnostic discrimination at age 3 to $3\frac{1}{2}$ years. Therefore, the SB-4 fails to differentiate among approximately the lowest 37% of children in the normal population.[24] Moreover, the lowest standard area score for quantitative reasoning up to $4\frac{1}{2}$ years of age is 72. For example, a raw score of 1 point on Bead Memory given to a 2-year-old child produces a standard score of 53 (slightly above average).[24] These floor limitations dissipate by age 5 to 6 years. Therefore, the test is best used at age 5 or older for children suspected of having developmental delays; reciprocally, the SB-4 has a good ceiling for gifted children (although gifted examinees score 20 points less on the SB-4 than the original SB).[23,24] The composite score averages 3 points lower than other IQ test scores (5 points < WISC-R, 3 points < WPPSI or PPVT-R). Correlations with the WISC-R range from $r = 0.02$ to 0.49.[25,26] However, the mean score differences changed depending on the child's ability level.[26–28] The SB-4 Composite is higher than the WISC-R at the lower end of the ability continuum but is lower than the WISC-R at the higher end. The two tests yield similar scores in the IQ 70 to 89 range.[27,28] Correlations with the Kaufman Assessment Battery for Children (K-ABC) are higher: $r = 0.68$ to $r = 0.89$.[24] The Binet Short-term Memory is best compared to the K-ABC Sequential Processing, Binet Abstract/Visual Reasoning with K-ABC Simultaneous Processing, and K-ABC Mental Processing Composite with the Binet Composite score.[24]

In summary, the technical properties of SB-4 are less impressive for preschool, as opposed to older children.[24,26,27] Greater bands of error affect test interpretation in younger children making it much less reliable. The test also does not contain the same subtests across applicable age ranges. The short-term memory factor appears appropriate for children aged 7 years and older.[27] The utility of the quantitative factor also is questionable.[27] Reciprocally, the test can be adapted to special populations: Nonverbal Reasoning/Visualization subtests are applicable for hearing-impaired children, whereas Verbal subtests can be grouped and used with children having visual impairments.[24] The abbreviated SB-4 batteries make the test useful as a screener or shortened version; the abbreviated batteries correlate with other measures of intelligence as highly as does the Test Composite.[27]

7.6. KAUFMAN ASSESSMENT BATTERY FOR CHILDREN

The Kaufman Assessment Battery for Children[29] (KABC) (Figure 7.4), developed in 1983, is a battery of tests applicable from ages $2\frac{1}{2}$ to $12\frac{1}{2}$ years. Usage has increased steadily over the last several years. In a recent survey of school psychologists, it was ranked second behind the WISC-R in terms of use (the Standard–Binet Form L-M and Stanford–Binet—Fourth Edition were third and fourth, respectively).[30] The test still is considered controversial by some, and interest warranted a special issue of the *Journal of Special Education*.[31]

The K-ABC is purported to measure two constructs: intelligence and achievement.[32] The test distinguishes sequential and simultaneous processing based on neuropsychological theory. Emphasis is placed on the

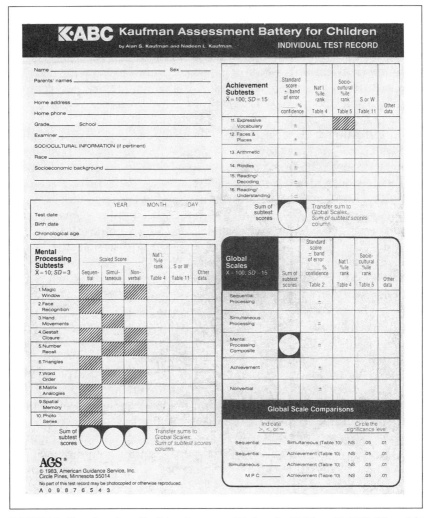

FIGURE 7.4. Face sheet from Kaufman Assessment Battery for Children (K-ABC). (Copyright 1983 American Guidance Service, Inc., 4201 Woodland Road, Circle Pines, MN 55014-1795. All rights reserved.)

process used to solve a problem (either linear/analytic/sequential or gestalt/ holistic/simultaneous) rather than the *content* of the task, as in the case of the WISC-R.[29],[31] Each task on the Sequential Processing Scale is solved by arranging the input in a sequential or serial order. This process is closely related to school-oriented skills such as memorization of number facts, lists of spelling words, phonics, grammatical rules, understanding sequences of events, and applying stepwise mathematics procedures such as borrowing. Problems included in the Simultaneous Processing Scale are spatial, analogic, or organizational in nature, with input being integrated and synthesized simultaneously to produce a solution. This process is related to tasks such as learning shapes of letters and numbers, deriving meaning from pictures (e.g., maps), acquiring a "sight" vocabulary, and comprehending text relationships. Essentially, these two processes broadly correspond to left- and right-hemispheric function.

The K-ABC yields a Sequential Processing standard score, a Simultaneous Processing standard score, a Mental Processing Composite, and an Achievement standard score (M = 100, SD = 15 for each). There are three sequential and seven simultaneous subtests, each with a mean of 10 (SD = 3). Not all of the tests are administered at each age level. Overall intellectual function is derived from a combination of the sequential and simultaneous scores into the Mental Processing Composite (which is intended to be a measure of total intelligence). In addition, the K-ABC contains six achievement scales that measure reading, arithmetic, general information, and language concepts. The achievement scales will not be discussed in detail in this section.

- *Sequential Tasks*. These tasks include (1) hand movements (requiring the child, aged $2\frac{1}{2}$ to $12\frac{1}{2}$ years to replicate a sequence of hand movements demonstrated by the examiner), (2) number recall (in which the $2\frac{1}{2}$- to $12\frac{1}{2}$-year-old child repeats a series of number sequences ranging from two to eight digits), and (3) word order (where the 4- to $12\frac{1}{2}$-year-old child points to sequences of pictures that correspond to series of words said by the examiner).
- *Simultaneous Tasks*. These tasks include (1) magic window (administered to children aged $2\frac{1}{2}$ to 4 years and requiring identification of an object such as a tree after viewing only a part), (2) face recognition (also given to $2\frac{1}{2}$- to 4-year-olds, in which the child identifies a previously seen face from a group photograph), (3) gestalt closure (the $2\frac{1}{2}$- to $12\frac{1}{2}$-year-old child must mentally fill in missing details of a partial drawing in order to identify an object such as bird), (4) triangles (two-colored triangle shapes are assembled into various abstract configurations by children aged 4 to $12\frac{1}{2}$ years), (5) matrix analogies (measures the 5- to $12\frac{1}{2}$-year-old child's ability to select the picture or design that best completes a visual analogy), (6) spatial memory (administered to children 5 to $12\text{-}\frac{1}{2}$ years, in which they recall the locations of pictures arranged randomly on a page), and (7) photo series (an array of photographs is organized to portray an event in chronological order by a 6- to $12\frac{1}{2}$-year-old child). The face recognition, hand movements, triangles, matrix analogies, spatial

memory, and photo series tests can be combined to produce a "nonverbal" score.[29] A short form of the K-ABC includes four tests: triangles, word order, matrix analogies, and hand movements.

The K-ABC tasks primarily are nonverbal, thereby making the test useful in the assessment of minority groups, bilingual children, and those with speech/language deficits or other learning disabilities. Verbal and factual items are more prevalent on the Achievement scales. Comparison between the Mental Processing Composite and levels of academic achievement is useful in the evaluation of learning disabilities, as is the use of the nonverbal scales to yield intelligence estimates in children with communication problems. Sequential/simultaneous discrepancies are also diagnostically useful. In children with learning disabilities, simultaneous processing standard scores typically are higher than sequential processing scores by 6 to 8 points; the Mental Processing Composite also is usually greater than Achievement Scale scores. An average simultaneous/sequential discrepancy of 13 points is significant at the $p < 0.05$ level, 18 points is significant at $p < 0.01$.[34]

The K-ABC produces only two meaningful factors before the age of 4 years: simultaneous and sequential. The achievement factor does not become relevant until age 4 and actually is most useful for school-aged children.[32] In children below age 4, the Expressive Vocabulary, Faces and Places, and Riddles are best interpreted as measures of simultaneous processing; Arithmetic is primarily a sequential subtest.[32] The test authors suggest that practitioners can gain insight into the nature of the preschool child's language problem by studying his/her performance on the Magic Window, Gestalt Closure, Expressive Vocabulary, Riddles, and Faces and Places subtests.[29,32] On these subtests, word-finding disorders (circumlocutions) often are evident in the child's tendency to describe a word instead of naming it[32] or giving the name of an object associated with the item being reviewed (e.g., "ring" versus "key" on the Riddles subtest).[32]

In at-risk preschoolers (age 49 to 73 months) evaluated two times over a 9-month interval, the Simultaneous Processing scale improved by almost 10 points, while the Sequential and Achievement scales improved by approximately 3 points. The Mental Processing Composite improved by an average of 8 points.[35]

As is the case with several other tests mentioned previously, there is a limited floor on several K-ABC subtests for very young or mentally retarded examinees. Moreover, there is an insufficient ceiling to challenge gifted children above 10 years of age. (Triangles and matrix analogies are considered the best subtests for gifted children.) The lack of assessment of expressive language is considered a drawback in testing preschoolers. The K-ABC correlates $r = 0.58$ to 0.91 with the WISC-R, depending on the nature of the sample (median = 0.84 with "normals"), r = 0.89 with the Stanford–Binet—Fourth Edition (this may be somewhat inflated), and r = 0.60 with the McCarthy Scales.[32-34] The K-ABC Mental Processing Composite typically will be several points lower than the WISC-R. Nonetheless, the K-ABC is a useful tool in the diagnostic evaluation of preschoolers, and it can differentiate normal children from handicapped and at-risk children. Practical application in the evaluation of hearing-impaired or language-impaired children is another attractive feature. However, practitioners should expect that the K-ABC Mental Processing scales will yield higher scores than other IQ tests in children with language problems. Conjoint use of the WISC-R or the WPPSI-R and the K-ABC provides an excellent evaluation of learning problems in school-aged children.

7.7. WIDE RANGE ASSESSMENT OF MEMORY AND LEARNING

The Wide Range Assessment of Memory and Learning[36] (WRAML), a new assessment instrument developed with a stratified sample of over 2300 subjects, was introduced in 1990. It is applicable for ages 5 to 17 years and is not a test of intelligence per se. Rather, the WRAML evaluates the child's ability to learn and memorize a variety of information. In actuality, these processes are a component of virtually every IQ test listed in Table 7.1. Since such abilities are intricately involved in IQ testing and school success, the WRAML was included in this chapter. This test is useful in assessment of learning disabilities, effects of head injury, and attention problems.

The WRAML has three components: (1) verbal memory, (2) visual memory, and (3) learning. The first two components involve remembering information and providing subsequent recall, whereas the learning scale involves the acquisition of new information over four trials. As a result, a Verbal Memory Index (VERI), Visual Memory Index (VISI), Learning Index (LRN), and a General Memory Index (derived from combination of the first three indices) are produced. Each index contains three subtests; the mean index score is 100 (SD = 15), whereas the mean subtest scaled score is 10 (SD = 3). Standard scores and percentiles are provided. In addition, the WRAML includes a delayed recall component (see Figure 7.5).

- *Verbal Memory Index*. This index involves rote memory in tasks of increasing semantic complexity. In Number/Letter Memory, the child repeats random combinations of numbers and letters (ranging from two to ten units). Sentence Memory requires the child to repeat meaningful sentences verbatim. In Story Memory, two short stories are read by the examiner, with the child recalling as many salient components as possible.

WRAML

**WIDE RANGE ASSESSMENT
OF MEMORY AND LEARNING**

EXAMINER FORM

NAME: _____ SEX: M F
SCHOOL: _____ GRADE: _____
REFERRED BY: _____ EXAMINER _____
DATE OF EXAM: YR. _____ MO. _____ DAY _____
BIRTHDATE: YR. _____ MO. _____ DAY _____
AGE: YR. _____ MO. _____ DAY _____

Subtests	Raw Score	Verbal	Visual	Learning
1. Picture Memory	____			
2. Design Memory	____			
3. Verbal Learning	____			
4. Story Memory	____			
5. Finger Windows	____			
6. Sound Symbol	____			
7. Sentence Memory	____			
8. Visual Learning	____			
9. Number/Letter	____			

Sum of Scaled Scores: ◯ ◯ ◯

WRAML Index Scores

Verbal Memory Index
(Sum of Verbal Scaled Scores) VERI
◯ • ☐ ____

Visual Memory Index
(Sum of Visual Scaled Scores) VISI
◯ • ☐ ____

Learning Index
(Sum of Learning Scaled Scores) LRNI
◯ • ☐ ____

General Memory Index
(Sum of all Scaled Scores) GMI
◯ • ☐ ____

Index   %ile

WRAML Scales — Scale Scores 1 2 3 4 5 6 7 8 9 10 11 12 13 14 15 16 17 18 19

Verbal Scale
Story Memory ☐
Sentence Memory ☐
Number/Letter Memory ☐
Verbal Memory Index — 70 · 85 · 100 · 115 · 130

Visual Scale
Picture Memory ☐
Design Memory ☐
Finger Windows ☐
Visual Memory Index — 70 · 85 · 100 · 115 · 130

Learning Scale
Verbal Learning ☐
Sound Symbol ☐
Visual Learning ☐
Learning Index — 70 · 85 · 100 · 115 · 130

Delayed Recall Subtests	Difference Scores	Level of Performance				
		Atypical	Borderline	Low Avg.	Average	Bright Avg.
Verbal Learning Recall	☐	◯	◯	◯	◯	◯
Story Memory Recall	☐	◯	◯	◯	◯	◯
Sound Symbol Recall	☐	◯	◯	◯	◯	◯
Visual Learning Recall	☐	◯	◯	◯	◯	◯
Story Memory Recog. Score	☐	◯	◯	◯	◯	◯

JASTAK
ASSESSMENT SYSTEMS

FIGURE 7.5. Face sheet from Wide Range Assessment of Memory and Learning (WRAML). (Copyright 1990 W. Adams & D. Sheslow. Reprinted with permission of the authors.)

- *Visual Memory Index*. This scale incorporates responses to increasingly meaningful visual material. Finger Windows involves replication of a visual sequential pattern in which the examiner places a pen in a series of holes on a card. In Design Memory, four designs are shown; after a 10-sec delay the designs are reproduced by the child. Picture Memory contains complex, meaningful scenes (e.g., beach) where the child views a picture for 10 sec and then looks at a second, similar scene and indicates alterations.
- *Learning Index*. Verbal Learning involves a list of 13 or 16 words (depending on age) that is recalled over four trials. The verbal learning curve is of interest, as it may provide clues as to whether the child has problems with attention or with verbal processing. In Visual Learning, a fixed number of stimuli are presented over four trials. Essentially, the child is required to remember the particular position of designs on a board, vis-à-vis the game "Memory." Sound Symbol is a paired association task in which the child recalls sounds that are associated with various abstract figures (e.g., two parallel lines might be associated with the sound "lex" as in "lexington"). This cross-modal task (verbal and visual) also contains four trials.

The Delayed Recall component contains four tasks: Verbal Learning, Visual Learning, Sound Symbol, and Story Memory. The WRAML takes approximately 45–60 min to complete; a 10- to 15-min screening version contains Picture Memory, Design Memory, Verbal Learning, and Story Memory. The 95% confidence interval for Verbal Memory is ±8, Visual Memory ±10, Learning ±9, and the General Memory Index ±6. The WRAML correlates with the WISC-R Full-Scale IQ ($r = 0.36$–0.56), MSCA Memory Index ($r = 0.72$), and SB-4 Short-Term Memory scale ($r = 0.80$).[36]

Clinically, the WRAML is particularly useful in detecting less-apparent learning problems such as a dysfunction in auditory processing (often seen as in poor performance on the Story Memory and Verbal Learning subtests) or difficulty in dual conceptual tracking (again observed on the Verbal Learning task and perhaps Number/Letter Memory). Poor performance on the Story Memory Task appears related to problems in reading comprehension. The physician should anticipate that this test most likely will be used on an increased basis over the next several years.

7.8. KAUFMAN BRIEF INTELLIGENCE TEST

The Kaufman Brief Intelligence Test[37] (K-BIT) is a new instrument that provides a quick measure of a child's intelligence. The test was normed on over 2000 individuals and is applicable for ages 4 to 90 years. Reliability and validity figures are quite acceptable. Administration of the K-BIT requires from 15 to 30 min, depending on age (e.g., for ages 4–7 years, 15 to 20 min is necessary; for children ages 8–19, 20 to 25 min is required). The instrument measures verbal and nonverbal intelligence by use of Vocabulary (Expressive Vocabulary and Definitions) and Matrices standard scores. In addition, an overall score, the "IQ Composite Standard Score," is produced by combining the Vocabulary and Matrices scores. The mean standard is 100 (SD = 15).

- *Vocabulary*. The 81-item vocabulary portion of the K-BIT consists of two parts. In the 45-item Expressive Vocabulary section, the child is required to provide oral responses by naming a pictured object such as a lamp or a calendar. Children ages 13 or older typically obtain a near-perfect score on this subtest. In the 37-item Definitions subtest (administered to children 8 years and older), two clues are provided, and the child must "guess" the correct word based on a verbal definition and a visual clue. For example, the examiner might say "a bright color," and the child would be presented with "YE_L_W" printed on the easel. The student then has to name the word. The Vocabulary standard score is thought to measure crystallized thinking, namely, word knowledge and verbal concept formation. As a result, this score is influenced by cultural/experiential influences arising from the home and school. Scores on the Expressive Vocabulary and Definitions subtests cannot be separated and compared.
- *Matrices*. Matrices contains 48 items that measure nonverbal skills and the child's ability to solve new problems. Fluid thinking, the child's ability to perceive relationships and complete analogies, is involved. Both meaningful (people and objects) and abstract (designs and symbols) stimuli are employed, and determination of relationships between the stimuli in a multiple-choice format is required. In the earlier items, the child must select which one of five pictures goes best with the stimulus picture, e.g., a car with a truck or a dog with a bone. Visual analogies are used as the items become more difficult; e.g., a hat goes with a head as a shoe goes with a foot. Later items use symbols and designs (see Figure 7.6). The Matrices subtest is considered to be more culture-free and therefore is useful in screening children from lower socioeconomic households. In addition, this subtest is helpful in the evaluation of children with special needs, such as those with motor or language problems.

Correlations between the Vocabulary and Matrices standard scores increase with age: $r = 0.44$ for ages 4–7; $r = 0.60$ for ages 8–19 years.[37]

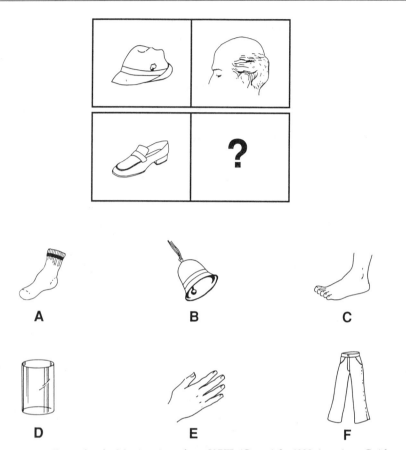

FIGURE 7.6. Example of a Matrices item from K-BIT. (Copyright 1990 American Guidance Service, Inc., 4201 Woodland Road, Circle Pines, MN 55014-1796. All rights reserved.)

Different starting points are recommended, depending on the child's age; confidence intervals are provided for each age. Descriptive categories, based on the Composite IQ score, are included: (1) average (90–109), (2) below average (80–89), (3) well below average (70–79), (4) lower extreme (<69), or (5) above average (110–119), (6) well above average (120–129), and (7) upper extreme (>130).

The K-BIT IQ Composite correlates fairly highly with the Kaufman Assessment Battery for Children (K-ABC) ($r = 0.58$–0.69) and the WISC-R Full-Scale IQ ($r = 0.80$).[37] However, the mean score difference between the K-BIT and WISC-R in the normative population is 5.9 points (the WISC-R being higher than the K-BIT). In a referred population, the correlation was almost identical to that of the standardization group ($r = 0.81$); however, the K-BIT Composite IQ was 6.2 points lower than the WISC-R FSIQ.[38] Similarly, the WISC-R Performance IQ was, on average, 8.3 points higher than the Matrices standard score, and the Verbal IQ was 2.9 points higher than the Vocabulary standard score.[38] More data are needed in regard to the relationship between the K-BIT and the WISC-III.

An attractive feature of the K-BIT is that it is not restricted to psychologists and can be administered by a variety of professionals. However, as the authors indicate, the K-BIT should not be a substitute for a comprehensive evaluation of a child's intelligence. The K-BIT provides a brief, gross measure of intelligence, but it does not yield a diagnosis. Rather, the test is a screening instrument that is useful when the practitioner is faced with significant time constraints.

REFERENCES

1. Wechsler, D., 1989, *Manual for the Wechsler Preschool and Primary Scale of Intelligence-Revised*, The Psychological Corporation, San Antonio.
2. Sattler, J. M., 1982, *Assessment of Children's Intelligence and Special Abilities*, ed. 2, Allyn and Bacon, Boston.
3. Gyurke, J. S., 1990, The assessment of preschool children with the Wechsler Preschool and Primary Scale of Intelligence—Revised, in: *The Psychoeducational Assessment of Preschool Children* (B. A. Bracken, ed.), Allyn and Bacon, Needham Heights, MA.
4. Bracken, B. A., 1992, Review of the Wechsler Preschool and Primary Scale of Intelligence—Revised, in: *The Eleventh Mental Measurements Yearbook* (J. J. Kramer and J. Close-Conoley, eds.), University of Nebraska Press, Lincoln.
5. The Psychological Corporation, 1989, *WPPSI-R. A Technical Report*, **1:**1–6.
6. The Psychological Corporation, 1990, *WPPSI-R. A Technical Report*, **2:**1–6.
7. Slate, J. R., and Saddler, C. D., 1990, The WPPSI-R: Comments and review. Improved but not perfect, *Natl. Assoc. School Psychol. Commun.* **Oct:**20.
8. Bracken, B. A., 1990, The WPPSI-R: Comments and review. Improved but not perfect. *Natl. Assoc. School Psychol. Commun.* **Oct:**21–22.
9. Wechsler, D., 1974, *Manual for the Wechsler Intelligence Scale for Children—Revised*, The Psychological Corporation, New York.
10. Wechsler, D., 1981, *Manual for the Wechsler Adult Intelligence Scale—Revised*, The Psychological Corporation, New York.
11. Kaufman, A. S., 1976, A four-test short form of the WISC-R, *Contemp. Ed. Psychol.* **1:**189–196.
12. Kaufman, A. S., 1979, *Intelligent Testing with the WISC-R*, John Wiley & Sons, New York.
13. Reynolds, C. R., and Kaufman, A. S., 1990, Assessment of children's intelligence with the Wechsler Intelligence Scale for Children—Revised (WISC-R), in: *Handbook of Psychological & Educational Assessment of Children* (C. R. Reynolds and R. W. Kamphaus, eds.), Guilford Press, New York.

14. Bannatyne, A., 1974, Diagnosis: A note on recategorization of the WISC scale scores, *J. Learn. Dis.* **1:**272–274.
15. Wechsler, D., 1991, *Wechsler Intelligence Scale for Children—Third Edition Manual*, The Psychological Corporation, San Antonio.
16. Flynn, J. R., 1987, Massive IQ gains in 14 countries. What IQ tests really measure, *Psychol. Bull.* **101:**171–191.
17. Hieronymus, A. N., and Hoover, H. D., 1986, *Iowa Tests of Basic Skills Form G*, Riverside Publishing, Chicago.
18. CTB/McGraw-Hill, 1988, *California Achievement Tests, Form E*, McGraw-Hill, Monterey, CA.
19. Prescott, G. A., Balow, I. H., Hogan, T. P., and Farr, R. C., 1986, *Metropolitan Achievement Test* (ed. 6), The Psychological Corporation, San Antonio.
20. Thorndike, R. L., Hagen, E. P., and Sattler, J. M., 1986, *Guide for Administering and Scoring the Fourth Edition. Stanford–Binet Intelligence Scale*, Riverside Publishing, Chicago.
21. Thorndike, R. L., Hagen, E. P., and Sattler, J. M., 1986, *Technical Manual. Stanford–Binet Intelligence Scale* (ed. 4), Riverside Publishing, Chicago.
22. Delaney, E. A., and Hopkins, T. F., 1987, *The Stanford–Binet Intelligence Scale: Fourth Edition. Examiner's Handbook*, Riverside Publishing, Chicago.
23. Glutting, J. J., and Kaplan, D. D., 1990, Stanford–Binet Intelligence Scale, Fourth Edition: Making the case for reasonable interpretations, in: *Handbook of Psychological and Educational Assessment of Children. Intelligence and Achievement* (C. R. Reynolds and R. W. Kamphaus, eds.), Guilford Press, New York, pp. 277–295.
24. McCallum, R. S., 1991, The assessment of preschool children with the Stanford–Binet Intelligence Scale: Fourth Edition, in: *The Psychoeducational Assessment of Preschool Children* (ed. 2) (B. A. Bracken, ed.), Allyn and Bacon, Boston, pp. 107–132.
25. Bracken, B. A., 1987, Limitations of preschool instruments and standards for minimal levels of technical adequacy, *J. Psychoed. Assess.* **5:**313–326.
26. McCallum, R. S., and Karnes, F. A., 1987, Comparison of the Stanford–Binet Intelligence Scale (4th ed.), the British Ability Scales, and the WISC-R, *School Psychol. Int.* **8:**133–139.
27. Laurent, J., Swerdlik, M., and Ryburn, M., 1992, Review of validity research on the Stanford-Binet Intelligence Scale: Fourth Edition, *Psychol. Assess.* **4:**102–112.
28. Prewett, P. N., and Matavich, M. A.,1992, Mean-score differences between the WISC-R and the Stanford-Binet Intelligence Scale: Fourth Edition, *Diagnostique* **17:**195–201.
29. Kaufman, A. S., and Kaufman, N. L., 1983, *Interpretive Manual for the Kaufman Assessment Battery for Children*, American Guidance Service, Circle Pines, MN.
30. Obringer, S. J., 1988, A survey of perceptions by school psychologists of the Stanford–Binet IV. Paper presented at the Meeting of the Mid-South Educational Research Association, Louisville, KY.
31. Miller, T. L., and Reynolds, C. R., 1984, The K-ABC [special issue], *J. Spec. Ed.* **18.**
32. Kamphaus, R. W., and Kaufman, A. S., 1991, The assessment of preschool children with the Kaufman Assessment Battery for Children, in: *The Psychoeducational Assessment of Preschool Children* (ed. 2) (B. A. Bracken, ed.), Allyn and Bacon, Boston, pp. 154–167.
33. Kamphaus, R. W., Kaufman, A. S., and Harrison, P. I., 1990, Clinical assessment practice with the Kaufman Assessment Battery for Children (K-ABC), in: *Handbook for Psychological and Educational Assessment of Children. Intelligence and Achievement* (C. R. Reynolds and R. W. Kamphaus, eds.), Guilford Press, New York, pp. 259–276.
34. Kamphaus, R. W., and Reynolds, C. R., 1987, *Clinical and Research Applications of the K-ABC*, American Guidance Services, Circle Pines, MN.

35. Lyon, M. A., and Smith, D. K., 1986, A comparison of at-risk preschool children's performance on the K-ABC, McCarthy scales, and Stanford–Binet, *J. Psychoed. Assess.* **4:**35–43.
36. Sheslow, D., and Adams, W., 1990, *Wide Range Assessment of Memory and Learning. Administration Manual,* Jastek Associates, Wilmington, DE.
37. Kaufman, A. S., and Kaufman, N. L., 1990, *Kaufman Brief Intelligence Test Manual,* American Guidance Service, Circle Pines, MN.
38. Prewet, P. N., 1992, The relationship between the Kaufman Brief Intelligence Test (K-BIT) and the WISC-R with referred students, *Psychol. School* **29:**25–27.

8 ❀ Assessment of Academic Achievement

8.1. INTRODUCTION

Interest in individually administered achievement tests has increased dramatically since the introduction of PL 94-142 [Education for All Handicapped Children Act, 1975, now entitled the Individuals with Disabilities Education Act (IDEA)]. A major reason for this increase is that these tests are a critical component in the diagnosis of learning disabilities (LDs) (Chapter 6). The testing instruments that will be described differ from group tests such as the Iowa Tests of Basic Skills[1] or the Stanford Achievement Test.[2] These latter tests are administered at specified times over the course of a child's school career.

Traditionally, it is assumed that individually administered tests of academic achievement will (1) identify children who need special instructional assistance, (2) help recognize the nature of a child's difficulties or deficiencies and thereby discriminate learning problems, and (3) assist in planning instruction and intervention.[3,4] However, it is questionable whether this type of testing adequately addresses these needs. First, it appears that the derived, norm-referenced information typically describes global achievement. Consequently, it may be less useful in diagnosing specific problems. Second, it has been suggested that teacher referrals may be the best indicator of those children who require special resource services. Third, low achievement test scores may be obtained by children with learning disabilities as well as by low-achieving regular classroom students. In addition, achievement testing also can be "unsettling" for a child who has a significant learning dysfunction. Frequently these children are highly sensitive to their area of difficulty. As a result, motivational issues, maladaptive test behavior, and the fact that testing typically terminates after the child has produced a string of failures are significant concerns. Furthermore, tests of academic achievement routinely are used simply to provide age- or grade-equivalent scores. Error analysis, which yields useful diagnostic information, typically is underemployed. Evaluation of the *types* and *patterns* of errors provides more important information regarding underlying dysfunctions and prescriptive data that are useful in planning intervention strategies.

The listing of tests of academic achievement that follows is not exhaustive. It represents those tests used most commonly and those with which primary-care physicians will have an increased probability of contact (see Table 8.1).

8.2. WIDE-RANGE ACHIEVEMENT TEST-REVISED

In a recent survey of psychological tests used in outpatient mental health facilities, the Wide Range Achievement Test-Revised (WRAT-R) was found to be the most frequently employed test of academic achievement.[6] This test instrument has undergone six revisions, the last occurring in 1984. (Another revision, the WRAT-3, will become available shortly.) The WRAT-R is very brief (a feature that has prompted criticism, yet reciprocally, also has served to enhance its popularity). The WRAT-R contains three subtests: reading (recognizing and naming letters, pronouncing words), spelling (copying marks that resemble letters, writing name, spelling words), and arithmetic (counting, reading numbers, solving oral and written problems). There are two levels: level I for age 5-0 through 11-11, and level II for ages 12 through 74-11. (The WRAT-3 will have two equivalent alternate test forms, each being used for individuals aged 5 through 74 years.) Grade ratings, standard scores ($M = 100$, $SD = 15$; range 46–155), and percentiles are provided. Grade ratings are arranged as "beginning," "middle," and "end of grade" for grades 1 and 2 and "beginning" and "end" for grades 3 through 12. Depending on the child's age, the test takes 15 to 30 min to administer.

The WRAT-R was standardized on a sample of 5600 individuals, although they were not stratified by socioeconomic status. The WRAT-R scores tend to be 8 to 11 points lower than the previous WRAT versions.

Advantages of the WRAT-R include: (1) it is a quick screen; (2) it is readily adaptable to primary-care office use; and (3) the youngest applicable age (5-0 years) is lower than that of many other tests of academic achievement. However, drawbacks include the lack of reading comprehension and arithmetic reasoning items as well as its focus on mechanics rather than conceptual knowledge. Since each child is compared to same-aged peers, a child who has repeated a grade is at a distinct disadvantage when his or her standard scores are computed, because the comparison will be made to same-aged peers who are a grade advanced.

TABLE 8.1. Tests of Academic Achievement

Test	Applicable grade/age	Date	Publisher	Administration	Level
Wide-Range Achievement Test-Revised (WRAT-R)	I. 5-0 to 11-11 II. 12 to 74-11 (grades K–12)	1984	Jastek Associates, Wilmington, DE	Various professionals	Screening
Basic Achievement Skills Individual Screener (BASIS)	6-0 to 18-11 (grades 1–12)	1983	The Psychological Corp., San Antonio, TX	Various professionals	Screening
Kaufman Test of Educational Achievement (KTEA)	6-0 to 18-11 (grades 1–12)	1985	American Guidance Service, Circle Pines, MN	Various professionals	Screening or comprehensive
Woodcock–Johnson Psycho-Educational Battery-Revised (WJ-R)	3-0 to 80+ (preschool– 12)	1989	DLM Teaching Resources, Allen, TX	Educators/psychologists	Comprehensive
Peabody Individual Achievement Test-Revised (PIAT-R)	5-3 to 18-11 (K–12)	1989	American Guidance Service, Circle Pines, MN	Various professionals	Screening
Boder Test of Reading/ Spelling Patterns	5-3 to adult (K–13)	1982	Grune & Stratton, New York	Various professionals	Screening/diagnosis reading
Wechsler Individual Achievement Test (WIAT)	5-0 to 19-11 (K–12)	1992	The Psychological Corp., San Antonio, TX	Various professionals	Screening or comprehensive

In general, as with many tests of academic achievement, grade ratings on the WRAT-R are problematic. Prior to the most recent revision, grade ratings were more detailed (e.g., prekindergarten, grade 1.1, 1.2, etc.). Perhaps in an effort to deemphasize the importance of such comparisons, the grade ratings were made more general. Grade scores also are problematic because there are no true national standards of instruction for each grade level. In addition, grade ratings are sometimes misused, as with repeated testing, increments in a grade rating are sometimes viewed as improvement scores. Reciprocally, however, grade ratings are not affected by having a child repeat a grade.

When reviewing or administering the WRAT-R, primary-care physicians should consider grade ratings, standard scores, and percentiles in combination. The data that are obtained are best viewed only as *screening* information, and consideration of the child's previous academic history (namely, repeating a grade) is necessary.

8.3. THE BASIC ACHIEVEMENT SKILLS INDIVIDUAL SCREENER

The Basic Achievement Skills Individual Screener[7] (BASIS), normed on 3300 children, is a "screener" used to assess reading, mathematics, and spelling for grades 1 to 12. In addition, the test includes an optional writing exercise. The BASIS takes 45 to 60 min to administer.

The reading section of the BASIS contains two readiness tests: letter identification and visual discrimination (in which the child views a group of letters—e.g., "name—and then must pick this grouping from an array of four similar groups of letters—e.g., "mame"). The reading test per se enables assessment of the child's comprehension of graded passages that are read aloud by means of the child pointing to the appropriate picture that depicts the sentence and by supplying missing word(s) in stories.

The mathematics section also includes a readiness component in which basic number concepts are evaluated ("less than," "more than," and counting). Additional problems are found in the test booklet and contain basic math functions such as addition, subtraction, multiplication, division, fractions, and decimals.

In the spelling subtest, six words are presented at each grade level; these are dictated by the examiner and then written by the student. In the writing section, the student is allowed 10 min to describe a favorite place. The passage is scored "average," "above average," or "below average" based on ideas, organization, vocabulary, sentence structure, and mechanics. Unfortunately, scoring is highly subjective.[8]

The BASIS has a mean (M) standard score of 100 (SD = 15), and percentile ranks, age equivalents, and grade placements can be derived. It correlates with report-card grades in the $r = 0.25$ to 0.61 range and with other achievement tests from $r = 0.50$ to 0.60. The BASIS ceilings out at approximately 14 years and therefore is best administered from ages 6 to 14 (approximately to grade 8). Usefulness with low-functioning younger students (e.g., slow first graders) is limited.[8] The interrater reliability for the writing test is questionable, and there is a need for some measure of silent reading.[8–10]

8.4. KAUFMAN TEST OF EDUCATIONAL ACHIEVEMENT

The Kaufman Test of Educational Achievement (KTEA) is available in two formats: the Comprehensive and Brief forms. In the former, reading decoding, reading comprehension, math application, math computation, and spelling are evaluated. In the Brief form, three areas are assessed: (1) reading (reading decoding and comprehension are combined), (2) math (math application and computation are combined), and (3) spelling. The test is administered to children in grades 1 to 12 (ages 6-0 to 18-11), and standard scores (M = 100, SD = 15), percentiles, stanines, and age and grade equivalents are provided. In addition, a battery composite score can be computed. The fact that a child can be compared to either same-aged or same-grade peers is an advantage. Moreover, this circumvents, to some degree, the problem that arises when a child has repeated a grade. In addition, fall and spring norms are provided, although the situation in which a child is at a cutoff month (e.g., August) sometimes is problematic. The Comprehensive form takes 60 to 75 min to administer, whereas the Brief form requires approximately 30 to 40 min (depending on grade). The Brief form is particularly useful for office screening and correlates highly ($r = 0.80–0.93$) with the Comprehensive form (see Figure 8.1).

The Brief form reading section includes letter and word identification and comprehension (in which the child mimes or answers verbally a short passage that he/she has read). Mathematics involves number computations and word problems. Spelling requires the child to spell dictated words.

Although very time efficient, the KTEA encounters problems with older children who have high achievement scores or younger children with significant academic delays. The highest score is 120, and therefore the ceiling for gifted children is limited. In addition, accurate assessment is difficult if a 6-year-old child is well below his/her grade or age level.[10] The lack of kindergarten norms is also a drawback at this time.

K-TEA

KAUFMAN TEST of EDUCATIONAL ACHIEVEMENT

by Alan S. Kaufman & Nadeen L. Kaufman

Brief Form

Individual Test Record

Student's Name _____ Sex _____

Parent's Name _____

Home Address _____

Home Phone _____

Grade _____ Teacher _____

School _____ Examiner _____

	Year	Month	Day
Test Date	_____	_____	_____
Birth Date	_____	_____	_____
Chronological Age	_____	_____	_____

BRIEF FORM SUBTESTS Mean = 100 SD = 15	Raw Score	Standard Score*	Band of Error ____% Confidence Table 5 or 6	%ile Rank Table 7	Other Data
MATHEMATICS		⬭	±		
READING		⬭	±		
SPELLING		⬭	±		
BATTERY COMPOSITE Mean = 100 SD = 15		▢	±		Descriptive Category

		AGE	GRADE
*STANDARD SCORES derived from (circle the table used):	Fall Norms (August–January)	Table 1	Table 2
	Spring Norms (February–July)	Table 3	Table 4

SUBTEST COMPARISONS (TABLE 10 or 11)

Indicate >, <, or ≈.

		Standard Score Difference	Circle the Significance Level
Mathematics	Reading		NS .05 .01
Mathematics	Spelling		NS .05 .01
Reading	Spelling		NS .05 .01

AGS®

8.5. WOODCOCK–JOHNSON PSYCHOEDUCATIONAL BATTERY-REVISED: TESTS OF ACHIEVEMENT

The Woodcock–Johnson Psychoeducational Battery[12] (WJ-R) contains Tests of Cognitive Ability, Tests of Interest Level, and Tests of Achievement. Although it is designed as a cohesive unit, the Tests of Achievement are often administered independently or in conjunction with other tests of intelligence. The Achievement Standard Battery, available in two parallel forms, contains nine subtests: letter–word identification, passage comprehension, calculation (mathematics), applied problems, dictation, writing samples, science, social studies, and humanities. Four subtests (letter–word identification, applied dictation, social studies, and humanities) are considered early developmental measures. Tasks in the Standard Battery include (1) identifying isolated letters and words, (2) reading a short passage and identifying a missing key word, (3) mathematics operations such as addition, subtraction, multiplication, and division, (4) practical math problems (e.g., counting the number of pencils in a picture), (5) spelling, punctuation, and dictation (contractions, capitalization), (6) writing responses to a variety of demands (e.g., "write a sentence that tells three things you study in school"), (7) biological and physical sciences (e.g., "name an insect that likes nectar"), (8) history, geography, and government, and (9) knowledge in art, music, and literature.

The nine subtests are grouped into five clusters: Broad Reading, Broad Mathematics, and Broad Written Language (each having two subtests), and Broad Knowledge, and Skills (each containing three subtests). The Skills cluster is considered an early developmental measure.

In addition, the WJ-R Tests of Achievement contain a Supplemental Battery consisting of word attack, reading vocabulary, quantitative concepts, proofing, and writing fluency. Functions assessed on this Supplemental Battery include phonic and structural analysis, synonyms and antonyms, knowledge of math concepts and vocabulary, identifying mistakes in typewritten passages, and formatting and writing simple sentences. These supplementary subtests are grouped into Reading, Mathematics, and Written clusters.

The WJ-R was normed on more than 6300 individuals aged 24 months to 95 years. Achievement testing begins at the preschool–kindergarten range. Psychometric aspects of the test are sound, and basal and ceiling rules are used. A variety of scores are obtained from the WJ-R Achieve-

FIGURE 8.1. Face sheet from the Kaufman Test of Educational Achievement (KTEA). (Copyright 1985 American Guidance Service, Inc., 4201 Woodland Road, Circle Pines, Minnesota 55014-1796. All rights reserved.)

ment data: standard scores (M = 100, SD = 15; range 40–160+), age and grade equivalents, and percentiles. In addition, there is the Relative Performance Index (RPI), which is the percentage of mastery predicted for an examinee when the reference group performs at a 90% level of success. The RPI is applied in a fashion similar to the Snellen Index to describe visual acuity; therefore, a 40/90 RPI means that where the reference group shows 90% mastery, the examinee is likely to demonstrate 40% mastery of specific subject matter. An instructional range band is also provided that indicates the range of tasks that a subject would perceive as quite easy (96% successful) to more difficult (75% successful).

At preschool ages, the WJ-R Achievement tests correlate well with other test instruments such as the Boehm Test of Basic Concepts (Chapter 4) and the Peabody Picture Vocabulary Test-Revised (r = 0.53 and 0.52, respectively). At school age, correlations in the r = 0.60 to 0.70 range were found with the BASIS, K-ABC achievement tests, K-TEA, Peabody Individual Achievement Test, and WRAT-R.[12]

The WJ-R Achievement tests require 30 to 45 min for administration, and the battery often is administered by special education teachers. However, scoring is intricate; in fact, an entire manual is devoted to scoring tables. Transferring data from these multiple tables increases the possibility of errors. Moreover, the array of scores can be overwhelming and confusing. Scores such as the "W" score (which is a transfer score) basically are of no use to the practitioner. Computer scoring programs are available, and these tend to minimize error problems. The time necessary for scoring is lengthy, and therefore the WJ-R is not practical for office use.

8.6. PEABODY INDIVIDUAL ACHIEVEMENT TEST-REVISED

The Peabody Individual Achievement Test-Revised[13] (PIAT-R), an extensive revision of the 1970 PIAT, contains six content areas: (1) General Information (100 items measuring general encyclopedic knowledge), (2) Reading Recognition (100-item oral test of reading), (3) Reading Comprehension (82 items in which a sentence is read silently and a picture is selected that best illustrates the sentence), (4) Mathematics (100 items involving mathematics concepts and facts), and (5) Spelling (a total of 100 readiness items and tasks requiring selection of correct spelling of words spoken by the examiner). All subtests are presented on easels, and not all items of any one subtest are administered to a child.

The General Information subtest contains 40% social studies items, 40% science, and 20% fine arts and humanities. The first 16 items of the Reading Recognition subtests involve analysis of early classroom reading materials by utilizing a pool of letter–sound items. Items 17 to 100 are single words read aloud. Analytic (look and say) and synthetic (phonics) approaches are balanced. Fifty percent of the mathematics items involve practical application of mathematics in everyday tasks and problems, 30% necessitate understanding of concepts, and 20% incorporate computational skills.[14] No reading is involved in the mathematics subtest.

In addition, a Written Expression subtest is included—with this being a significant new feature. The Written Expression subtest contains two levels: level I is applicable for kindergarten and first grade (child copies letters, words, and sentences or writes from dictation); level II is appropriate for grades 2 to 12 (student is given 20 min to write a story in response to a picture prompt). The Written Expression task is particularly useful in the evaluation of processing problems as outlined in PL 94-142 (Chapter 6). Grade-based stanines are available for both levels I and II, whereas a developmental scaled score is available for level II. However, scoring for level II is more subjective than for level I.[14] The PIAT-R yields two Composite Scores: Total Reading (consisting of reading recognition and reading comprehension) and a Total Test Score (consisting of the first five subtests).

The PIAT-R (which retains only 35% of the items from the original PIAT) was standardized on 1563 individuals and contains norms for grades K through 12 and ages 5-0 to 18-11. Testing takes approximately 60 to 75 min. Basal and ceiling ages are used, with items being arranged in order of ascending difficulty. Grade equivalents, age equivalents, standard scores ($M = 100$, $SD = 15$; range 55 to 145), percentile ranks, normal curve equivalents, and stanines are produced. The normal curve equivalents ($M = 50$; $SD = 21.06$) are used in reporting Chapter 1 evaluations to the federal government.

The PIAT-R correlates moderately well with total test scores of other achievement tests such as the WRAT-R and the PIAT ($r = 0.62$–0.88 range); correlation with the K-ABC achievement tests is higher ($r = 0.86$).[13] Scores on the PIAT-R tend to be 6 to 8 points lower than scores obtained with the original PIAT. The PIAT-R incorporates many items with multiple-choice formats and thereby involves recognition versus recall. For example, instead of simply spelling a word, the child is asked to choose the dictated word from four printed alternatives. This format is used in Mathematics and Reading Comprehension as well. As a result, scores on the PIAT-R may be higher than those obtained with other tests because of this multiple-choice format.

The PIAT-R could be used in an office setting, particularly if only selected subtests were utilized. The Written Expression component is very helpful in the evaluation of learning disabilities, particularly since it adopts an analytical approach with different writing components being scored (e.g., thoughts expressed in complete sentences, appropriate verb tense, correct pronoun usage, meaning is understandable). The pediatrician should be cognizant of the fact that the PIAT-R is a screening instrument and therefore should not be used as a diagnostic tool in isolation. Moreover, it is more sensitive to academic difficulties in lower grades (i.e., up to fourth grade) than in later grades.[14] The PIAT-R's design (i.e., no writing or use of pencils) enables testing of children who are physically handicapped.

8.7. BODER TEST OF READING–SPELLING PATTERNS

The Boder Test of Reading-Spelling Patterns[15] is designed specifically to aid in the diagnosis of reading problems, which often are grouped under the term "dyslexia." It is a useful clinical instrument that readily is applicable to office administration. The Boder enables analysis and classification of the *types* of errors found in a child's reading and spelling performance; it addresses the issue of error analysis mentioned in the introduction of this chapter.

The basic premise of the Boder Test is that there are two components involved in the reading process: the visual gestalt and the auditory-analytic. The former involves sight vocabulary, visual perception, and memory for whole words; the latter incorporates word-analysis skills. Based on test results, the Boder enables classification of children with reading problems into three groups: (1) dysphonetic (unable to integrate written symbols with sounds, thereby having problems with phonic word analysis; e.g., "even" spelled as "evernt," "child" as "chilly"), (2) dyseidetic (problems with the visual gestalt, but with intact phonics skills; e.g., "laugh" spelled as "laff," "order" as "ordr," "was" as "saw," or "tool" as "loot"), and (3) mixed dysphonetic–dyseidetic (displaying characteristics of both disorders).

On the Boder, the child is required to read progressively more difficult word lists consisting of 20 words (one-half phonetic, one-half nonphonetic). Lists begin at a primer level, and the child continues until six or fewer words out of a 20-word list are read correctly. On the spelling component, a list of 10 words previously read correctly (five phonetic, five nonphonetic) and a list of 10 words not read correctly (with the same phonetic/nonphonetic split) are presented.

The examiner evaluates differences in spelling and reading errors, differences in spelling phonetic and nonphonetic words, and other clinically relevant indicators that are outlined in the manual.[15] A reading quotient (RQ) is also produced (RQ = reading age/chronological age × 100).

Advantages of the Boder Test include its diagnostic potential, simplicity, and applicability in regard to prescriptive suggestions. The reading quotient and lack of normative data detract from its use as an indicator of age or grade levels for reading. It is recommended that the Boder be used in conjunction with other achievement tests listed in this chapter to allow for a more thorough assessment of reading problems.

8.8. WECHSLER INDIVIDUAL ACHIEVEMENT TEST

The Wechsler Individual Achievement Test[16] (WIAT) is the newest individually administered achievement battery. It was designed for the assessment of children in grades kindergarten through 12 (aged 5 years to 19 years 11 months). The WIAT was normed on more than 4500 individuals, with the mean standard score being 100 (SD = 15) and scores ranging from 40 to 160. Age- and grade-based standard scores, percentiles, stanines, and normal curve equivalents are provided in addition to age and grade equivalents.

The Comprehensive WIAT contains eight subtests (Figure 8.2); three of the subtests, Basic Reading, Mathematics Reasoning, and Spelling, can be used as a brief Screener. The Comprehensive battery requires 30 to 50 min administration time for young children and approximately 55 min for adolescents; the Screener necessitates 10 to 20 min for administration. Practitioners can expect a 30- to 50-min testing period for children in kindergarten through second grade; 55 to 60 min is required for those in grades 3 through 12 (without administration of the written expression subtest).

According to the authors,[16] the WIAT is unique in that it is the only achievement test directly linked with the Wechsler Intelligence Scales. By conorming the WIAT in conjunction with the WISC-III, WPPSI-R, and WAIS-R (see Chapter 7), "linked data" are provided. These data enable examiners to calculate meaningful aptitude–achievement discrepancies in the diagnosis of learning disabilities (see Chapter 6). In addition, the WIAT also includes several unique areas of assessment: Oral Expression, Listening Comprehension, and Written Expression. The subtests are as follows:

- *Basic Reading.* A series of pictures and printed words are presented to assess decoding skills (phonetic analysis and word analysis) and word-reading abilities. In the early items, the child is requested to point to a word that has the same beginning or ending sound as the picture. Later items require the child to read words aloud.

WIAT™
WECHSLER INDIVIDUAL ACHIEVEMENT TEST™

Record Form

Summary

Child's Name ______ Sex ____
School ______ Grade ____
Teacher ______ Examiner ______
Referral Source ______
Reason for Referral ______

	Year	Month	Day
Date Tested			
Date of Birth			
Age			

Behavioral Observations ______

WIAT Subtests

☐Age ☐Grade

	Raw Scores				Standard Score	Confidence Interval ___%	Percentile	Other ____ ☐ Equivalent ☐ NCE
Basic Reading						–		
Mathematics Reasoning						–		
Spelling						–		
Reading Comprehension						–		
Numerical Operations						–		
Listening Comprehension						–		
Oral Expression						–		
Written Expression						–		

Composites

☐Age ☐Grade

	Reading	Mathematics	Language	Writing	Total Composite
Sum of Raw Scores	+	+	+	=	
Standard Score					
Confidence Interval ___%	–	–	–	–	–
Percentile					
Other ____ ☐Equivalent ☐NCE					

THE PSYCHOLOGICAL CORPORATION®
HARCOURT BRACE JOVANOVICH, INC.

09-972076

FIGURE 8.2. From the Wechsler Individual Achievement Test (WIAT). (Copyright 1992 by The Psychological Corporation. Reproduced by permission.)

- *Mathematics Reasoning.* This subtest includes counting, basic computations, word problems, and other mathematics reasoning tasks (measurement, numeration, comparing decimals and fractions). Many items involve visual stimuli (e.g., graphs, geometric figures). Each item is presented verbally by the examiner, and the child may respond verbally or can write his/her response on paper. This subtest measures mathematics abilities that are beyond routine computational skills.
- *Spelling.* A series of dictated letters, sounds, and words are presented verbally, and the child must write his/her responses. The test measures encoding and spelling ability with words that require regular and irregular spellings. Homophones (words pronounced alike but spelled differently) comprise 10% of the items (e.g., "to" versus "two," "ate" versus "eight").
- *Reading Comprehension.* The child is presented with a passage of one or more sentences (some accompanied by pictures), which he/she reads. The examiner then asks specific questions about the passage, and the child must respond verbally. Skills such as making inferences, comparing and contrasting, and recognizing stated detail are measured.
- *Numerical Operations.* In this subtest, the child is presented with written mathematics problems (at earlier ages, writing down dictated numbers is required). Calculation of problems and solving equations involving addition, subtraction, multiplication, division, fractions, decimals, and introductory algebraic equations are involved.
- *Listening Comprehension.* Initial items assess the child's ability to identify (by pointing) the picture that corresponds to an orally presented word (receptive vocabulary). Later items involve the examiner reading a passage to the child and subsequently asking questions about the passage. Comprehension of verbally presented material is tapped.
- *Oral Expression.* This subtest contains a series of items that focus on the child's ability to express words, describe scenes, give directions, and describe a sequence of steps required to complete a task (e.g., how to purchase a soda from a machine). So-called "pragmatics" of language (i.e., informing, instructing, explaining) are evaluated.
- *Written Expression.* The child is required to write a hypothetical letter in response to a prompt (e.g., describe how you would like your ideal house to look). Development and organization of ideas, grammar, capitalization, and punctuation are scored for children in grades 3 through 12. This subtest allows direct evaluation of a child's written discourse; however, it is the most difficult subtest to score.

As is evident in Figure 8.1, the Reading Composite, Mathematics Composite, Language Composite, and Writing Composite summary scores each contain two subtests. In regard to time requirements, Mathematics Reasoning, Reading Comprehension, and Listening Comprehension are the longest subtests.[16] If the examiner is faced with time limitations, Reading Comprehension, Numerical Operations, and Written Expression can be used in conjunction with the Screener to provide information on the three basic achievement areas.

Correlations between the WIAT and the BASIS[7] range from $r = 0.79$ to 0.84 for reading and 0.75 to 0.85 for mathematics. In regard to the KTEA,[11] correlations with the WIAT are high ($r = 0.86$ for reading recognition, 0.87 for mathematics, and 0.78 for reading comprehension). In general, KTEA standard scores are 3 to 9 points higher than the corresponding WIAT scores. Correlations between the WRAT-R[5] and WIAT are also fairly high: reading, $r = 0.84$; numeric operations, 0.77; and spelling, 0.84. Little difference exists between the standard scores. Comparison of scores between the WIAT and Woodcock–Johnson Psychoeducational Battery-Revised[12] also revealed strong associations ($r = 0.67$–0.88), although the WIAT standard scores generally were several points lower than those of the WJ-R.

Comparison of the WIAT Listening Comprehension subtest and the PPVT-R revealed substantial correlations ($r = 0.75$), as did comparison of the PPVT-R and the WIAT Reading and Reading Comprehension subtests ($r = 0.68$). Correlations with group-administered subtests also were significant.

WIAT raw scores can be compared to age or grade norms (fall, winter, and spring comparisons in the case of grade). Tables are provided that allow prediction of WIAT subtest and composite scores from WISC-III full-scale IQs. Additional tables contain differences between predicted and actual scores that are necessary for statistical significance.

In summary, outstanding features of the WIAT include ability–achievement comparisons, ease of administration and interpretation, and inclusion of the Oral Expression and Listening Comprehension subtests (which are attractive in LD evaluations).[17] A table of skills analysis for each of the subtests also is provided, thereby enabling practitioners to determine "patterns" of deficit.

Drawbacks of the WIAT include the fact that starting levels sometimes are altogether too easy for average or above-average students, yet the "floor" often is too high at lower ages for children with poorly developed readiness skills.[17] The latter circumstance makes it difficult to document a severe discrepancy in this younger group. In addition, because the Written

Language composite contains both Spelling and Written Expression subtests, strengths or weaknesses in either of these areas may affect the composite score and cause erroneous interpretation. The WIAT Screener is particularly useful for the practitioner.

8.9. SUMMARY

The preceding discussion focuses on individual rather than group achievement tests such as the Gates–MacGinitie Reading Tests-Third Edition,[18] California Achievement Tests,[19] Comprehensive Tests of Basic Skills,[20] Iowa Tests of Basic Skills,[1] or the Stanford Achievement Test.[2] These group-administered tests typically are used by school systems to ascertain teaching effectiveness and to determine a child's grade levels and areas of strength and weakness. Virtually all of these group tests measure various components of reading, language, spelling, and mathematics. Study skills, science, social studies, and listening also are evaluated on some. As a result, these tests are referred to as multilevel survey batteries (see Nitko and Lane[21] for a more detailed discussion), and they cover more material than individually administered achievement tests.

In summary, individual achievement testing is necessary whenever the primary-care physician is faced with the child who demonstrates academic difficulties. These tests may also be used as a quick screen in children presenting with recurrent physical complaints for which no organic basis can be found, behavior problems (particularly refusal to do school work), or suspected attention-deficit disorders. Often these problems are secondary to a child's inability to perform adequately in the classroom environment because of an underlying learning problem. Nonetheless, this type of evaluation should be considered as a screening only, because individually administered achievement tests merely measure global accomplishment in academic areas.

Finally, achievement-testing data must be compared to a child's performance on intelligence tests, particularly in cases where there might be a discrepancy between verbal and performance scores. For example, if a child obtains a low WISC-R (or WISC-III) verbal IQ and a high performance IQ, the child might be at a "double disadvantage" because he/she missed the prerequisite verbal abilities necessary for academic learning. Basing classroom achievement expectancies on the high performance IQ may not be realistic.[22] Therefore, analysis of a comprehensive achievement-testing profile in conjunction with intelligence measures is essential.

REFERENCES

1. Hieronymus, A. N., Linquist, E. F., and Hoover, D., 1984, *Iowa Tests of Basic Skills*, Riverside Publishing, Chicago.
2. Gardner, E. F., Rudman, H. C., Karlsen, B., and Merwin, J. C., 1984, *The Stanford Achievement Test Series*, Psychological Corporation, New York.
3. Goetz, E. T., Hall, R. J., and Fetsco, T. G., 1990, Implications of cognitive psychology for assessment of academic skill, in: *Handbook of Psychological and Educational Assessment of Children. Intelligence and Achievement* (C. R. Reynolds and R. W. Kamphaus, eds.), Guilford Press, New York.
4. Salvia, J., and Ysseldyke, J. E., 1988, *Assessment in Special and Remedial Education* (ed. 4), Houghton Mifflin, Boston.
5. Jastek, S., and Wilkenson, G. S., 1984, *Wide Range Achievement Test-Revised*, Jastek Associates, Wilmington, DE.
6. Piotrowski, C., and Keller, J. W., 1989, Psychological testing in outpatient mental health facilities: A national study, *Prof. Psychol. Res. Pract.* **20**:423.
7. Psychological Corporation, 1983, *Basic Achievement Skills Individual Screener Manual*, Psychological Corporation, San Antonio.
8. Huebner, E. S., 1984, Test review: Basic Achievement Skills Individual Screener (BASIS), *J. Psychoed. Assess.* **2**:173–176.
9. Sattler, J. M., 1988, *Assessment of Children* (ed. 3), Jerome M. Sattler, San Diego.
10. Kamphaus, R. W., Slotkin, J., and DeVincentis, C., 1990, Clinical assessment of children's academic achievement, in: *Handbook of Psychological and Educational Assessment of Children. Intelligence and Achievement* (C. R. Reynolds and R. W. Kamphaus, eds.), Guilford Press, New York.
11. Kaufman, A. S., and Kaufman, N. L., 1985. *Kaufman Test of Educational Achievement*, American Guidance Service, Circle Pines, MN.
12. Woodcock, R. W., and Johnson, M. B., 1989, *Woodcock–Johnson Psycho-Educational Battery-Revised*, DLM Teaching Resources, Allen, TX.
13. Markwardt, F. C., 1989, *Peabody Individual Achievement Test-Revised*, American Guidance Service, Circle Pines, MN.
14. Luther, J. B., 1992, Review of the Peabody Individual Achievement Test-Revised, *J. School Psychol.* **30**:31–39.
15. Boder, E., and Jarrico, S., 1982, *The Boder Test of Reading–Spelling Patterns*, Grune & Stratton, New York.
16. Psychological Corporation, 1992, *Wechsler Individual Achievement Test Manual*, Psychological Corporation, San Antonio.
17. Sharp, A., 1992, The WIAT: Evaluation of assessment for provision of services under the Individuals with Disabilities Education Act (IDEA), *Child Assess. News.* **2**:8–10.
18. MacGinitie, W. H., and MacGinitie, R. K., 1989, *Gates MacGinitie Reading Tests* (ed. 3), Riverside Publishing, Chicago.
19. CTB Macmillan/McGraw-Hill, 1987, *California Achievement Tests*, Author, Monterey, CA.
20. CTB Macmillan/McGraw-Hill, 1990, *Comprehensive Tests of Basic Skills*, Author, Monterey, CA.
21. Nitko, A. J., and Lane, S., 1990, Standardized multilevel survey achievement batteries, in: *Handbook of Psychological and Educational Assessment of Children. Intelligence and Achievement* (C. R. Reynolds and R. W. Kamphaus, eds.), Guilford Press, New York.
22. Humphries, T., and Bone, J., 1993, Use of IQ criteria for evaluating the uniqueness of the learning disability profile, *J. Learn. Dis.* **26**:348–351.

9 ❋ Attention/ Concentration

9.1. DIAGNOSTIC ISSUES IN ATTENTION-DEFICIT DISORDERS

Attention-deficit disorders (ADD) can influence behavior, academic performance, and social and emotional adjustment. Problems in attention and concentration therefore should be considered routinely in the diagnostic evaluation of difficulties in school achievement. Unfortunately, many symptoms of ADD are relatively nonspecific; as a result, differential diagnosis is problematic. Attention deficits may co-occur, share common symptoms with, or overlap other disorders. Co-occurrence with oppositional/defiant and conduct disorders, anxiety/affective disorders, pica, Tourette syndrome, and learning disabilities is relatively frequent.[1] In fact, approximately 50% of children with ADD manifest symptoms that warrant the diagnosis of oppositional disorder, 70% of those with Tourette syndrome have attention deficits, and the prevalence of ADD among patients with learning disabilities ranges from 10% to 40%.[2] Symptoms similar to ADD often occur in mental retardation, pervasive developmental disorders such as autism, and among patients with speech/language disorders.[1]

The distinction between ADD with and without hyperactivity is highly controversial. This distinction is of particular significance for the practitioner who is evaluating problems in school performance. The DSM-III-R[4] espoused a "polythetic," unidimensional definition of ADD (termed attention-deficit hyperactivity disorder). However, combining symptoms has not been supported empirically.[5,6] This approach may obscure cases in which the attention deficit is the primary etiology for poor school performance.

Conceptualization of two types of ADD, a cognitive and a behavioral form, may help clarify this issue.[2] The cognitive type is associated with academic problems, inattention, impulsivity, and difficulty with information processing. The cognitive type, analogous to ADD without hyper-activity, is associated with a greater incidence (40–60%) of learning problems in mathematics and reading.[7,8] It also is associated with a "sluggish" cognitive tempo,[9] shyness, tendency to withdraw, anxious behavior, higher probability of repeating a grade, and a codiagnosis of anxiety or affective disorder.[9] Reports from teachers generally are more sensitive to this problem than are reports from parents.[10]

The behavioral type of ADD is more common than the cognitive form. Features of the behavioral form include inattention, impulsivity, hyper-activity, and frequent conduct disorders. This form (perhaps reflective of ADD with hyperactivity) usually is associated with more externalizing behaviors, less likelihood of grade retention, more frequent peer difficulties, fewer learning disabilities, and a codiagnosis of conduct disorder.[10–12] Children displaying ADD without hyperactivity are more likely to be referred to pediatricians, child neurologists, and psychologists because of problems in attention and learning. On the other hand, children with ADD and hyperactivity (particularly with aggressive components) routinely are referred to mental health centers and child psychiatrists.[13,14] Analyses of measurement data further support this dichotomy by identifying two dimensions of ADD: inattention–disorganization (cognitive) and motor hyperactivity–impulsivity (behavior).[5] The DSM-IV includes ADD with and without hyperactivity as distinct diagnoses. These are termed: Attention-Deficit/Hyperactivity Disorder: (1) Combined type (ADHD), (3) Predominantly Inattentive Type, and (3) Predominantly Hyperative-Impulsive Type.[15]

The "pervasive" versus "situational" classification of ADD may be related to the aforementioned distinction between ADD with and without hyperactivity. Children with pervasive ADD exhibit more severe symptoms, accompanied by hyperactivity and externalizing behaviors that occur across situations. Students with situational ADD often are of the cognitive type, with symptoms exaggerated by factors related to settings and particular tasks. Situations with low environmental demands are less likely to elicit symptoms than would reading or mathematics activities, complex assignments, or other tedious, sustained tasks.[11,16] Stressful environmental and psychosocial conditions and/or some medications (antihistamines, phenobarbital) can produce "hyperactive" behaviors that may be mistaken for ADD.

9.2. EVALUATION OF ATTENTION/CONCENTRATION

The diagnostic issues outlined above underscore the need for a comprehensive clinical assessment in children with suspected problems in attention and concentration. In addition to the techniques that follow, the assessment of children with attention deficits routinely begins with in-depth interviews of the parent(s) and the child[17] to ascertain whether or not certain diagnostic criteria are met.[4]

Techniques used in the clinical evaluation of problems in attention and concentration can be grouped into three areas: (1) rating scales, (2) instruments for evaluating specific aspects of ADD (impulsivity, attention, distractibility), and (3) psychometric measures of intelligence, academic achievement, memory, or processing. Many of these techniques formerly were regarded as laboratory measures,[18] but, during the last several years, their application in clinical settings has increased dramatically.

9.2.1. Rating Scales

Problems in attention and concentration are difficult to diagnose in pediatric offices.[19] Therefore, the use of adjunctive information sources has been emphasized.[20] As a result, a plethora of parent and teacher rating scales have evolved. Some rating scales are specific to attention-deficit disorders, whereas others evaluate broad-band emotional and behavioral problems. Content areas differ despite the fact that many scales are labeled in a similar fashion or are purported to deliberate similar patterns of deviant behavior.[21] Potential sources of confusion include how the scales are worded, the number of items used to measures specific constructs, whether the degree of the problem behavior can be measured, scale length, and psychometric issues such as reliability, validity, and availability of normative data.[22]

An in-depth description of rating scales used most frequently in the assessment of attention-deficit disorders is found in Chapter 10.

9.2.2. Instruments That Evaluate Specific Aspects of ADD

9.2.2.1. Computerized Assessment

There is increasing clinical application of computerized assessment devices in the evaluation of problems in attention and concentration.[23] Attention is a multidimensional concept that includes alertness and the ability to be selective or focused, to search, and to inhibit distractibility and impulsivity.[24] Therefore, instruments that evaluate specific aspects of this concept are of particular interest. The Continuous Performance Task[25] (CPT) and its variants[26–30] have been the mainstay in this line of investigation.

Although many versions of the CPT have been developed, in the basic procedure, the child responds to a specific letter, number, or combination of these symbols that is included within a sequence of irrelevant symbols (e.g., an "X"). The target symbol is preceded by a cue. The number of *correct responses* (accurate responses to target stimuli), *omissions* (target stimuli that are missed), and *commissions* (incorrect responses to irrelevant stimuli) are recorded. In existing CPT procedures, many different target stimuli are used: light pairs, numbers, letters, visual stimuli (shapes), and letters and colors. Task lengths vary from 4.75 to 30 min, and different stimulus durations are used (0.125 to 0.5 sec). Although there are at least 11 CPT versions currently available, several of the most frequently used clinical computerized assessment techniques are outlined below.

9.2.2.2. Gordon Diagnostic System

Perhaps the most widely used computerized procedure is the Gordon Diagnostic System[27] (GDS). The GDS is a portable microprocessor-based unit developed specifically for clinical use. The GDS contains three components: (1) a delay task (that requires a child to inhibit responding in order to earn points), (2) a vigilance task (CPT), and (3) a distractibility task (CPT with distractors). The GDS was normed on over 1300 children (see Figure 9.1).

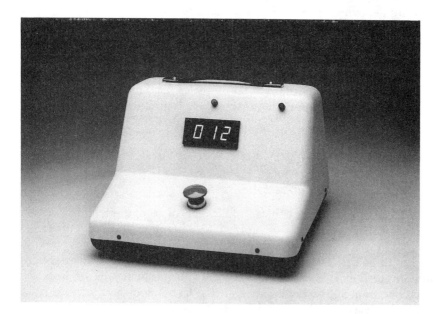

FIGURE 9.1. The Gordon Diagnostic System. (Reprinted with permission, GSI Publications.)

On the delay task, the child is requested to press a button, wait a short interval, and then press the button once again. If the child refrains from responding for at least 6 sec and then presses the button, a light flashes and a counter displays increments on a screen. If the child responds too quickly, the timer resets, and no reward points are recorded. The task takes 12 min (four 3-min blocks). The Efficiency Ratio (number correct/total number of responses) is the most useful indicator. This task is considered to measure impulsivity in a differential reinforcement of low-rate responding (DRL) procedure. The delay task is unique to the GDS and is not found in other computerized assessments.

The vigilance task is a CPT in which the child is requested to press the button every time a "1" is followed by a "9." The number correct, number of omissions (not responding to target stimuli), and the number of commissions (responding to irrelevant stimuli) are recorded. Each digit is displayed for a 0.2-sec period followed by a 1-sec interstimulus interval. The vigilance task consists of three 3-min trials and is considered to measure both attention and impulsivity. The distractibility task is identical to the vigilance task, with the addition of numbers (distractors) flashing on both sides of the center (target) stimuli. This task is also 9 min in duration and measures attention, impulsivity, and distractibility. Norms are available for preschool children through age 16 years.

9.2.2.3. Test of Variables of Attention

The Test of Variables of Attention[29] (T.O.V.A.) (formerly called the Minnesota Computer Assessment) is a 23-min computerized assessment. Whenever the "correct" stimulus is presented, the subject presses a firing button. One of two stimuli appears at various points on the screen for 100 msec every 2 sec. The designated target is presented on 22.5% of the trials during the first half of the test and on 77.5% of the trials during the second half (stimuli are colored squares containing a small square adjacent to either the top or bottom edge of the screen). This technique is non-language-based and requires no right–left discrimination. Norms are available for ages 5 years and older. Errors of omission, commission, reaction time, variability, and postcommission reaction time are derived. The T.O.V.A., available for Apple IIe and IBM PC-compatible computers, is considered to be a useful measure of inattention and impulsivity in clinical settings.

9.2.2.4. Conners Continuous Performance Test

The new Conners CPT "standard" administration[30] differs from most other versions. On this test, the child is required to press the appropriate key for any letter *except* "x." This technique assesses the child's ability to inhibit responding. The test contains 18 blocks of 20 trials, with the interstimulus interval being 1, 2, or 4 sec. The stimulus is presented for 250 msec. The entire test requires 14 to 16 min for administration. A very attractive feature of the Conners CPT is that it easily can be altered by the examiner to create new paradigms. A "regular" CPT procedure (responding to the target stimulus) also is provided.

Number of omissions, number of commissions, mean "hit" reaction time (mean time in milliseconds taken to respond correctly to target letters), mean commission reaction time, and total mean reaction time data are available. The availability of reaction time data is another positive feature.

On the Conners CPT, the "normal" rate for errors of omission is 1% to 2%; commissions should be less than 30%.[30] Reaction times greater than 900 msec are considered "sluggish," whereas the combination of fast reaction times and multiple commissions is considered to be indicative of impulsive responding.[30]

The normative sample size (293 individuals) is somewhat problematic, as only 25 children were used between 4 and 6 years of age, whereas 37 subjects provided normative data in the 16- to 18-year age range. In addition, although it is an intriguing concept, the utility of having a child *not* respond to target stimuli needs further evaluation.

9.2.2.5. Summary of Computerized Assessment

There are several general considerations regarding computerized assessment. Commission errors (responding to nontarget stimuli) do not appear to be homogeneous; commissions with fast reaction times reflect impulsivity, whereas those with slow reaction times are indicative of inattention. Commission errors also increase when response demands correspondingly become more difficult, and there often is an increase in errors of commission following an omission.[31,32] Children with high rates of responding often obtain a high number correct by virtue of probability; therefore, an Accuracy Index (which considers simultaneously the number correct and number of commissions, penalizing a child for the latter)[33] is recommended.

Age and intelligence appear to influence CPT performance, with older and more intelligent children obtaining better scores.[23] Brighter children with attention problems still may score in the normal range on these tasks. Moreover, sensitivity rates of CPT procedures in adolescents have been as low as 20%. Visual processing and visual memory deficits also can negatively affect CPT performance, and there are few good similar auditory measures available at this time. It appears that arousal affects the initial level of CPT performance, but it does not account for a decline in vigilance over time. As the interstimulus interval increases, the number of correct responses decreases. Children with attention-deficit disorders often perform poorly at both the fastest and slowest event rates. Therefore, presenting target stimuli at one speed (event rate) may miss some clinical cases. Moreover, inattention on the CPT can be a nonspecific problem for a number of psychiatric disorders.[34] The vigilance task commission measure is most sensitive to drug responses[35,36]; however, errors of omission, response time, and response variability have also been found to improve when psychostimulants are administered to children with ADD and to controls. There appears to be little practice effect on the CPT; in fact a *negative* practice effect exists in which a decline in performance results from the child being faced with a repetitive and boring task. Improvement therefore is attributable to *real* change and not just a practice effect.[30]

Some children do poorly on the GDS vigilance task but not on the distractibility task, suggesting the possibility of hypoarousal. In addition, there is evidence to suggest that the examiner's presence can affect a child's performance on the GDS. Children's ability to differentiate target stimuli from distractors is significantly worse during examiner absence than when he/she is present.[37] Clearly, computerized assessments should not be used in isolation but, rather, in conjunction with other sources of information.[11,21]

9.3. OTHER MEASURES

Several other techniques occasionally are utilized in the evaluation of problems in attention and concentration. Most of these techniques are used in research applications; however, they may prove to have clinical utility.

9.3.1. Matching Familiar Figures Test

The Matching Familiar Figures Test[38] (MFFT) is a measure of inhibitory control and has long been considered a "primary index" of impulsivity. The MFFT contains 12 tasks, each with a stimulus picture (e.g., a cat) and an array of six additional pictures, one being identical to the stimulus picture. The child (aged 5–11) selects a picture from the array of very similar pictures until the identical one is chosen. Errors and initial response latencies are recorded for each task and then are averaged. Error measures are more reliable than are the response latencies. A reportedly more reliable MFF-20[39] has been developed for ages 7 to 11 years. However, the utility of the MFFT has not been established for adolescents.

9.3.2. Children's Embedded Figures Test

The Children's Embedded Figures Test[40] (CEFT) was designed originally as a paper-and-pencil test of field dependence (finding a shape within an array of lines and shapes) and is considered a "measure of personality . . . designed to assess cognitive styles"[41] (p. 87). However, this test has been used as a measure of distractibility in ADD evaluations. Although potentially useful, the validity of the 25-item CEFT as a measure of attention and distractibility is questioned.

In general, the utility of these and similar tests has not been documented, limiting their use in clinical practice. Low between-test intercorrelations are a major issue, perhaps because these tests measure very circumscribed functions.[17] Additional instruments can be found in a review article by Brown.[18]

9.4. PSYCHOMETRIC TECHNIQUES

Psychometric techniques fall into two broad categories: tests of intelligence (Chapter 7) and tests of academic achievement (Chapter 8). In addition to providing information on specific aspects of attention disorders, these measures are necessary because of the high incidence of learning disabilities found in children with problems of attention and concentration. Although discrepancies between IQ and levels of academic achievement are considered indicators of learning disabilities (Chapter 6), problems in attention and concentration also can produce lower scores on either measure. As mentioned previously, available intelligence tests yield somewhat different information; all have the advantage of allowing for behavioral observation under standardized conditions (see Chapter 7).

The Wechsler Intelligence Scale for Children—Revised (WISC-R)[42] and the new WISC-III[43] are the most frequently used tests to assess intelligence. On the WISC-R, three factors are produced[44]: (1) verbal comprehension, (2) perceptual organization, and (3) freedom from distractibility (FFD). The freedom from distractibility factor (consisting of arithmetic, digit span, and coding) is often used in the evaluation of attention problems; however, its utility is questioned. The FFD factor most likely measures attention, concentration, sequencing ability, test anxiety, short-term memory, numerical or quantitative ability, and executive processing.[45] In addition to difficulties in any one of these areas, auditory processing difficulties, visual–motor integrative problems, or dyscalculia can produce a positive finding and therefore mimic attention problems. Reciprocally, children with attention-deficit problems may not obtain low scores on this factor because of associated strengths.

As was noted previously (Chapter 7), on the WISC-III, factor analyses revealed that the third factor (FFD) contains only two subtests, namely, arithmetic and digit span.[43] Coding does not load on FFD factor as it did on the WISC-R. The coding subtest, together with the new symbol search subtest, adds a fourth factor, "Processing Speed." As indicated previously (Chapter 7), the 45-item symbol search subtest requires that a child check off "yes" or "no" as to whether a specific symbol appears in a string of three to five corresponding symbols. In addition to IQ scores, four norm-referenced index scores, corresponding to the four factors, are now available. Comparison of these index scores is highly promising in the diagnosis of problems in attention and concentration.

The Wechsler Preschool and Primary Scales of Intelligence—Revised (WPPSI-R) contains several subtests helpful in the evaluation of problems in attention and concentration: (1) mazes, (2) animal pegs (a speeded matching task in which the child matches different colored pegs to pictures of animals, based on a key), (3) arithmetic, and (4) sentence recall. Scores on these subtests can be compared to other verbal and performance tasks to determine whether attention is an area of concern.

The Stanford–Binet—Fourth Edition (SB-4) contains a Short-Term Memory area score that includes memory for bead configurations, sentences, digits, and pictures of objects. Performance on these subtests and the overall area score can be compared to other subtests and area scores (see Chapter 7).

As noted previously (Chapter 7), the Kaufman Assessment Battery for Children[48] (K-ABC) yields sequential and simultaneous processing scores. The sequential scores are particularly sensitive to attention problems and include replication of a series of hand movements demonstrated by the examiner, number recall, and word order (child points to a series of pictures corresponding to words spoken by the examiner). The hand movement subtest seems particularly useful in assessing attention problems.

The Wide-Range Assessment of Memory and Learning[49] (WRAML) also aids in the evaluation of attention problems. There is evidence to suggest that the verbal memory tasks of sentence memory and number/letter memory (where the child repeats back auditory information) and the design memory and finger windows visual memory subtests (where the child draws previously viewed designs after a 10-sec delay and reproduces visual sequences demonstrated by the examiner by placing a finger in holes) are particularly sensitive to attention problems.[50] Separating WRAML tasks into: (1) strategic versus nonstrategic processing and (2) episodic versus semantic memory may help in ADD evaluation. In particular, children with ADD would be expected to experience more problems with nonstrategic, episodic tasks (rote) such as number/letter memory than with more semantic tasks (story memory).[51]

Tests of academic achievement provide insight into the types of errors a child makes, consistency of performance, and how problems in attention and concentration may affect classroom performance (see Chapter 8). Careless errors, inconsistency in performance, poor organization, or rapid deterioration in performance are particularly suggestive of attention problems.

9.5. INTERRELATIONSHIPS BETWEEN MEASURES

There tends to be little commonality between diagnostic measures of attention and concentration used in clinical populations. In a recent study of correlational analyses of checklists, computerized measures, and psychometric assessments, significant within-cluster correlations were found (i.e., checklists correlated with checklists, computerized assessment measures were related to other computerized assessment measures, etc.). However, between-cluster correlations were not significant, indicating that measures involving similar functions cluster together; those that assess different areas do not.[44] Moreover, parent rating scales, teacher checklists, and computerized assessment measures were in agreement (all indicating a positive or negative finding) in only 25% to 30% of cases.

Parent checklists appear too liberal in regard to indicating problems in attention and concentration, particularly if hyperactivity also is present. Computerized assessment is much more conservative, whereas teacher ratings fall between these two extremes.[52,53]

In summary, clinicians should be aware that reliance on a single diagnostic measure or a one-time evaluation is not recommended. A combination of diagnostic instruments is essential in order to determine adequately whether a child with poor school performance has difficulty with attention and concentration. Each diagnostic instrument measures specific aspects or functions of attention and concentration, and children with attention-deficit disorders form a heterogeneous population.[11]

Therefore, a protocol consisting of parent and teacher checklists, computerized assessment, and psychometric testing should be employed in this evaluation. An assessment model, outlined by Kelly and Aylward,[11] is found in Figure 9.2. This model lists the various components of an

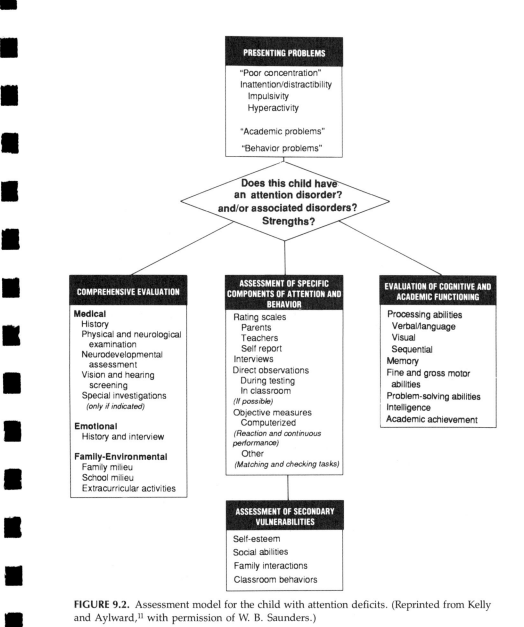

FIGURE 9.2. Assessment model for the child with attention deficits. (Reprinted from Kelly and Aylward,[11] with permission of W. B. Saunders.)

overall comprehensive evaluation of the child who presents with school problems.

REFERENCES

1. Cantwell, D. P., and Baker, L., 1987, Differential diagnosis of hyperactivity, *J. Dev. Behav. Pediatr.* **8:**159–165.
2. August, G. J., and Garfinkel, B. D., 1989, Behavioral and cognitive subtypes of ADHD, *J. Am. Acad. Child Adoles. Psychiat.* **28:**739–748.
3. Cantwell, D. P., and Baker, L., 1991, Association between attention deficit–hyperactivity disorder and learning disorders, *J. Learn. Dis.* **24:**88–95.
4. American Psychiatric Association, 1987, *Diagnostic and Statistical Manual of Mental Disorders* (3 ed., revised), American Psychiatric Association, New York.
5. Lahey, B. B., Pelham, W. E., Schaughency, E. A., Atkins, M. S., Murphy, H. A., et al., 1988, Dimensions and types of attention deficit disorder, *J. Am. Acad. Child Adoles. Psychiat.* **27:**330–335.
6. Hinshaw, S. P., 1987, On the distinction between attention deficits/hyperactivity and conduct problems/aggression in child psychopathology, *Psychol. Bull.* **101:**443–464.
7. Hynd, G. W., Lorys, A. R., Semrud-Clikeman, M., Nieves, N., et al., 1991, Attention deficit disorder without hyperactivity: A distinct behavioral and neurocognitive syndrome, *J. Child. Neurol.* **6:**37–42.
8. August, G. J., and Garfinkel, B. D., 1990, Comorbidity of ADHD and reading disability among clinic-referred children, *J. Abnorm. Child Psychol.* **18:**29–45.
9. Lahey, B. B., Schaughency, E. A., Hynd, G. W., Carlson, C. L., and Nieves, N., 1987, Attention deficit disorder with and without hyperactivity: Comparison of behavioral characteristics of clinic-referred children, *J. Am. Acad. Child Adoles. Psychiat.* **26:**718–723.
10. Lahey, B. B., and Carlson, C. L., 1991, Validity of attention deficit disorder without hyperactivity: A review of the literature, *J. Learn. Dis.* **24:**110–120.
11. Kelly, D. P., and Aylward, G. P., 1992, Attention deficits in school aged children and adolescents: Current issues and practice, *Pediatr. Clin. North Am.* **39:**487–512.
12. Goodyear, H. P., and Hynd, G. W., 1992, Attention deficit disorder with (ADD/H) and without (ADD/WO) hyperactivity: Behavioral and neuropsychological differentiation, *J. Clin. Child Psychol.* **21:**273–305.
13. Epstein, M. A., Shaywitz, S. E., Shaywitz, B. A., and Woolston, J. L., 1991, The boundaries of attention deficit disorder, *J. Learn. Dis.* **24:**78–86.
14. Loney, J., and Milich, R., 1982, Hyperactivity, inattention, and aggression in clinical practice, *Adv. Dev. Behav. Pediatr.* **3:**113–147.
15. American Psychiatric Association, 1994, *Diagnostic and Statistical Manual of Mental Disorders, Fourth Edition*, American Psychiatric Association, Washington, DC.
16. Barkley, R. A., 1990, A critique of current diagnostic criteria for attention deficit hyperactivity disorder: Clinical and research implications, *J. Dev. Behav. Pediatr.* **11:**343–352.
17. Barkley, R. A., 1991, Diagnosis and assessment of attention deficit–hyperactivity disorder, *Comp. Ment. Health Care* **1:**27–43.
18. Brown, R. T., 1982, Hyperactivity: Assessment and evaluation of rating instruments, *J. Psychiatr. Treat. Eval.* **4:**359–369.
19. Sleator, F. K., and Ullman, R.A., 1981, Can the physician diagnose hyperactivity in the office? *Pediatrics* **67:**13–17.
20. Blondis, T. A., Accardo, P. J., and Snow, J. H., 1989, Measures of attention deficit. Part I. Questionnaires, *Clin. Pediatr.* **28:**222–228.

21. Shaywitz, S. E., Shaywitz, B. A., Schnell, C., and Towle, V. R., 1988, Concurrent and predictive validity of the Yale Children's Inventory: An instrument to assess children with attention deficits and learning disabilities, *Pediatrics* **81**:562.

22. Barkley, R. A., 1981, *Hyperactive Children: A Handbook for Diagnosis and Treatment*, Guilford Press, New York.

23. Aylward, G. P., Verhulst, S. J., and Bell, S., 1990, Individual and combined effects of attention deficits and learning disabilities on computerized ADHD assessment, *J. Psychoed. Assess.* **8**:497–508.

24. Barkley, R. A., 1988, Attention, in: *Assessment Issues in Child Neuropsychology* (M. G. Tramontana and S. R. Hooper, eds.), Plenum Press, New York, pp. 145–176.

25. Rosvold, H. E., Mirsky, A. F., Sarason, I., Bransome, E. D., and Beck, L. H., 1956, A continuous performance test of brain damage, *J. Consult. Psychol.* **20**:343–350.

26. Conners, C. K., 1985, The computerized continuous performance test, *Psychopharmacol. Bull.* **21**:891–892.

27. Gordon, M., 1983, *The Gordon Diagnostic System*, Gordon Systems, Boulder, CO.

28. Swanson, H. L., 1983, A developmental study of vigilance in learning-disabled children, *J. Abnorm. Child Psychol.* **11**:415–429.

29. Greenberg, L. M., 1991, *The Test of Variables of Attention (T.O.V.A.)*, University Attention Disorders, Los Alamitos, CA.

30. Conners, C. K., 1992, *Continuous Performance Test Manual*, Multi-Health Systems, North Tonawanda, NY.

31. Conners, C. K., and Rothschild, G. H., 1968, Drugs and learning in children, in: *Learning Disorders*, Volume 3 (J. Hellmuth, ed.), Special Child Publications, Seattle, pp. 192–223.

32. Halperin, J. M., Sharma, V., Greenblatt, E., and Schwartz, S. T., 1991, Assessment of the continuous performance test: Reliability and validity in a nonreferred sample, *Psychol. Assess.* **3**:603–608.

33. Aylward, G. P., Verhulst, S. J., Bell, S., Kelly, D., and Dorry, G., 1988, The relationship between the GDS and DSM-III diagnoses: Introduction of the Accuracy Index (AI), *ADHD/Hyperact. Newslett.* **11**:2–4.

34. Halperin, J. M., Matier, K., Bedi, G., Sharma, V., and Newcorn, J. H., 1992, Specificity of inattention impulsivity, and hyperactivity to the diagnosis of attention-deficit hyperactivity disorder, *J. Am. Acad. Child Adol. Psychiat.* **31**:190–196.

35. Solanto, M. V., and Conners, C. K., 1982, A dose–response and time–action analysis of autonomic and behavior effects of methylphenidate in attention deficit disorder with hyperactive children, *Psychophysiology* **19**:658–667.

36. Barkley, R. A., and Edelbrock, C., 1987, Assessing situational variation in children's problem behaviors: The home and school situations questionnaires, in: *Advances in Behavioral Assessment of Children and Families*, Volume 3 (R. J. Prinz, ed.), JAI Press, Greenwich, CT, pp. 157–176.

37. Power, T. J., 1992, Contextual factors in vigilance testing of children with ADHD, *J. Abnorm. Child Psychol.* **20**:570–593.

38. Kagan, J., 1965, Reflection-impulsivity: The generality and dynamics of conceptual tempo, *J. Abnorm. Psychol.* **71**:17–24.

39. Cairns, E., and Cammock, T., 1978, Development of a more reliable version of the "Matching Familiar Figures Test," *Dev. Psychol.* **14**:555–560.

40. Karp, S. A., and Konstadt, N., 1987, *Children's Embedded Figures Test*, Consulting Psychologists Press, Palo Alto, CA.

41. Morgan, R. R., 1988, *Children's Embedded Figures Test*, Test Corporation of America, Kansas City.

42. Wechsler, D., 1974, *Manual for the Wechsler Intelligence Scale for Children—Revised*, The Psychological Corporation, New York.

43. Wechsler, D., 1991, *The Wechsler Intelligence Scale-III Manual*, The Psychological Corporation, New York.
44. Kaufman, A. S., 1979, *Intelligent Testing With the WISC-R*, John Wiley & Sons, New York.
45. Weiss, L. G., 1991, WISC-III: The Revision of the WISC-R, *Child Assess. News.* 1:1–9.
46. Wechsler, D., 1988, *WPPSI-R Manual*, Psychological Corporation, San Antonio.
47. Thorndike, R. L., Hagan, E. P., and Sattler, J. M., 1986, *Guide for Administering and Scoring the Fourth Edition Stanford–Binet Intelligence Scale*, Riverside Publishing, Chicago.
48. Kaufman, A. S., and Kaufman, N. L., 1983, *Interpretive Manual for the Kaufman Assessment Battery for Children*, American Guidance Service, Circle Pines, MN.
49. Sheslow, D., and Adams, W., 1990, *Wide-Range Assessment of Memory and Learning Administration Manual*, Jastek Associates, Wilmington, DE.
50. Aylward, G. P., Verhulst, S. J., and Bell, S., 1992, Relationship between measures of memory and attention: ADD or LD? Paper presented at the 1992 Convention of the American Psychological Association, Washington, DC.
51. Aylward, G. P., Verhulst, S. J., Bell, S., 1993, Interrelationships between measures of attention deficit disorders: Same scores, different reasons, *J. Dev. Behav. Pediatr.* 14:282.
52. Aylward, G. P., Kelly, D. P., Verhulst, S. J., and Bell, S., 1989, Diagnostic dilemmas in attention deficit disorders: Concordance between different assessment techniques, *J. Dev. Behav. Pediatr.* 10:274.
53. Cohen, M. L., Kelly, P. C., and Atkinson, A. W., 1989, Parent, teacher, child: A trilateral approach to attention deficit disorder, *Am. J. Dis. Child.* 143:1229–1233.

10 ❀ Behavioral Assessment

10.1. INTRODUCTION

In addition to evaluation of intelligence and achievement, assessment of emotional status and behavioral functioning is critical in the evaluation of school problems. Questionnaires, rating scales, and behavioral checklists are very useful in meeting this need in clinical pediatrics.[1] Information about the child's behavior at home and in school is essential in the diagnostic formulation. Rating scales are better than teacher interviews or classroom observations because of reduced time requirements, better organization of data, better cost efficiency, and the opportunity to compare children from a norm-based perspective.[2] Rating scales also add information not routinely observable in an office setting. However, a survey by the American Academy of Pediatrics revealed that only 45% of the respondents in general pediatric practice routinely used questionnaires.[3]

The terms "questionnaire," "rating scale," and "checklist" often are used interchangeably. Generally, checklists require a binary or discrete decision regarding a specific behavior (e.g., yes/no, present/absent). Rating scales, however, require that a behavior be rated on a scale containing three to nine points (e.g., little–much, seldom–frequent). Several instruments, such as the School Situations Questionnaire[4] or the Eyberg Child Behavior Inventory,[5] contain both components: behavior is rated as a problem (yes/no) and then is scored on a seven- to nine-point scale to indicate the severity of the problem. In keeping with the terminology of other reviews, the terms questionnaire, rating scale, and checklist will be used interchangeably.[1]

Questionnaires can be used for history taking, record keeping, or assessing parents' concerns about their child's behaviors. However, the questionnaires to be reviewed involve screening behaviors, quantifying behavioral information, assisting diagnosis, and evaluating treatment effects (as in the case of attention-deficit disorders).

The Likert Scale is the primary format used with rating scales. Here, a statement is followed by a series of graded responses with three to ten categories such as "strongly agree" to "strongly disagree," or "never" to "almost always." The reliability and validity of a scale increase when more than two anchor points are present.[6] Short scales are more likely to be completed than longer scales.

Eisert et al.[1] suggest that three types of reliability are important when questionnaires are used in primary-care settings: (1) *interrater reliability*— the degree to which different raters agree in their responses, such as agreement between parents and teachers, (2) *test–retest reliability*—the extent to which ratings made by the same rater at two different times agree, and (3) *split-half reliability*—a measure of internal consistency within a test, indicating the degree to which all test items measure the same dimension (see Chapter 1). Because of behavioral inconsistencies in children, temporary changes, and practice effects, the reliability values of checklists and rating scales often are not as high as would be desirable. In a recent review of a sample of 14 behavioral rating scales, approximately one-third had acceptable normative data that were both current and representative of the U.S. population.[2] This weakness also would have a negative effect on reliability. Moreover, because of the phenomenon of regression towards the mean (tendency for extreme scores to become less extreme when measured a second time), reports of problem behaviors tend to decrease whenever an instrument is measured a second time.[7] It has been suggested that reliability values of 0.50 for all three reliability types cited above are acceptable for questionnaires. This value is considerably lower than those for test instruments.

Validity, the degree to which a questionnaire measures what it is intended to measure, is also a concern (see Chapter 1). Four types of validity are particularly important when one is considering rating scales and questionnaires: (1) *content validity* (the extent to which the questionnaire items are representative of the pool of items measuring a certain behavior), (2) *construct validity* (whether the questionnaire measures a specific psychological construct such as attention), (3) *discriminant validity* (questionnaire's ability to discriminate between groups such as hyperactive versus not hyperactive, or constructs such as hyperactive versus oppositional), and (4) *criterion-related validity* (agreement between the questionnaire and other measures of the same behavior). A questionnaire that is valid for one population or setting may not be appropriate with other children or situations. In addition, readability, scoring issues, completion time, and norms must be considered. Clinicians *should not* attempt to make a diagnosis based on questionnaires. An excellent review on the use of questionnaires in behavioral pediatrics is provided by Eisert et al.[1]

Rating scales can measure emotional functioning and personality, characteristic behaviors (e.g., attention or activity), and/or adaptive functioning. They may vary by applicable age group, informant, setting, or types of classification provided. Discussion of rating emotional functioning and personality characteristics is beyond the purview of this chapter. Adaptive functioning is addressed in Chapter 4. The focus of this section is on problems in school functioning; therefore, the rating scales reviewed will involve instruments specific to attention-deficit disorders ("narrow-band") and others that sample more "broad-band" behaviors. Both types of rating scales have advantages and disadvantages, and both can be used by the practitioner. Broad-band measures allow for a wider sampling of behaviors such as withdrawal, anxiety, depression, delinquency, or aggression[8]; narrow-band measures are more restricted in the type of behavior that is evaluated, such as attention or hyperactivity. Broad-band factors are more reliable than narrow-band factors, and they allow clustering of children into groups on the basis of factor profiles. Narrow-band factors typically measure specific problems that are of interest to clinicians.[9]

10.2. RATING SCALES THAT MEASURE ATTENTION-DEFICIT PROBLEMS (UNIDIMENSIONAL)

As was indicated in the preceding chapter, attention-deficit problems (ADD) are difficult to diagnose in pediatric settings.[10] Therefore, the use of adjunctive informational sources has been recommended.[11] As a result, interest in parent and teacher rating scales has flourished. Some of these rating scales are *narrow-band* and specific to ADD, whereas others evaluate *broad-band* emotional and behavioral dimensions. Content areas often differ, even though many scales are labeled the same or are purported to describe similar patterns of deviant behavior.[12] Potential sources of confusion include wording of the scales, the number of items used to measure specific constructs, whether the *degree* of the problem can be measured, scale length, and psychometric issues such as reliability, validity, and availability of normative data.[13] Basically, not all rating scales are created equal.[14]

The reviews of rating scales that follow are not exhaustive; they represent instruments that the practitioner will encounter most frequently and that also provide the most useful information. These instruments generally are grouped into *parent* and *teacher* questionnaires.

10.2.1. Parent Rating Scales

Parents generally are perceived as being less reliable and less objective informants than teachers; however, they have had significantly longer contact with the child in a broader range of situations. Parents, as a rule, have a better understanding of situational aspects of the child's behavior. Multidimensional (broad-band) parental report measures discriminate ADD children from others more accurately than unidimensional, more specific instruments (narrow-band), perhaps because of the overlap between ADD and other behavioral and psychiatric problems (e.g., oppositional–defiant, anxiety, depressive, or conduct disorders).[15] Therefore, parent rating scales obviously complement those of teachers. The most prominent parent rating scales are listed in Table 10.1 and are described briefly in the following sections.

10.2.1.1. Conners Parent Rating Scale

The Conners Parent Rating Scale[16–18] (CPRS) is the most frequently used parent scale. Applicable from ages 3 to 17 years, the CPRS originally contained 93 items, but the revision consists of 48.[19] There is some debate concerning the scale's evolution.[20] Although the wording of different versions varied, scoring remained the same. The CPRS-48 contains five scales: (1) conduct problem, (2) learning problem, (3) psychosomatic, (4) impulsive–hyperactive, and (5) anxiety. In addition, a ten-item Hyperactivity Index, sometimes called the Conners Abbreviated Symptom Questionnaire (ASQ)—which is particularly sensitive to drug effects—is provided. Males generally score higher than females on the CPRS. Hyperactivity scores decrease as the child gets older. An increased anxiety scale score is related to decreased responsiveness to medication.[13] T-scores are provided with the new manual, and scores >70 are considered clinically significant. Ratings between mothers and fathers differ somewhat, with agreement ranging between 0.46 and 0.57.[19] On the CPRS, items such as "excitable, impulsive" or "fails to finish things" are scored 0 to 3 (not at all, just a little, pretty much, very much).

10.2.1.2. CLAM Questionnaire

A hybrid, 16-item (Conners, Loney, and Milich, CLAM) Questionnaire[21] has been developed. The CLAM consists of a combination of the Conners ten-item hyperactivity questionnaire and the Loney and Milich 15-item IOWA–Conners Questionnaire[22] (see Section 10.2.2.). There are four subscales: (1) a Conners hyperactivity index (scores >14 being significant), (2) an IOWA–Conners mixed inattention/overactivity and aggression/defiance factor, (3) an IOWA inattention/overactivity factor (>7 being significant), and (4) an IOWA aggression/defiance factor (>4). Items such as "restless or overactive" or "disturbs other children" are scored on a four-

TABLE 10.1. Parent Rating Scales

Scale	Ages/grades	Number of items	Type of assessment	Teacher form available	Publisher
Conners Parent Rating Scale (CPRS)	3–17 years	48	Narrow-band	Y	MultiHealth Systems
Conners, Loney, and Milich Questionnaire (CLAM)	K–5	16	Narrow-band	Y	Authors
Yale Children's Inventory (YCI)	K–5	11	Narrow-band	Y	Authors
Swanson, Nolan, and Pelham Rating Scale (SNAP)	6–11 years K–5	23	Narrow-band	Y	Authors
Self-Control Rating Scale (SCRS)	?	33	Narrow-band	N	Authors
Child Behavior Checklist (CBCL)	4–16 years	138	Broad-band	Y	University of Vermont
Revised Behavioral Problems Checklist (R-BPC)	5–17 years K–12	89	Broad-band	Y	Author
Aggregate Neurobehavioral Student Health and Education Review (ANSER)	4–6 years/6–11 years/12+ years	270	Broad-band	Y	Educators Publishing Service
Home Situations Questionnaire (HSQ)	4–18 years	16	Narrow-band	Y	Author
Children's Attention and Adjustment Survey (CAAS)	5–13 years K–5	31	Narrow-band	Y	American Guidance Serivce
Attention Deficit Disorders Evaluation Scale (ADDES)	4.5–18 years	46	Narrow-band	Y	Hawthorne Educational Service

point scale: "not at all" to "very much." This questionnaire presently is used more in research, rather than in clinical settings; however, it has clinical utility.

10.2.1.3. DSM-III-Based Checklists

Two checklists incorporate criteria from the American Psychiatric Association's *Diagnostic and Statistical Manual III* (DSM-III): *The Yale Children's Inventory*,[23] and the *Swanson, Nolan and Pelham (SNAP) Rating Scale*.[24] The former contains 11 behavioral and cognitive scales, including attention, hyperactivity, and impulsivity; the latter is normed for grades K to 5. On the SNAP, items such as "excessive running or climbing" are rated "not at all," "just a little," "pretty much," or "very much." Unfortunately, these rating scales are useful, but they do not correspond to criteria outlined in DSM-III-R or the new DSM-IV. Therefore, their future applicability may be limited. There is a 46-item SNAP-R, which also includes items from the DSM-III-R as well as several other sources[21]; however, usage is not widespread at present.

10.2.1.4. Self-Control Rating Scale

The 33-item Self-Control Rating Scale[25] (SCRS) is a unidimensional scale measuring a narrower band of behavior, namely, impulsivity/self-control. The SCRS, rated from 1 (always) to 7 (never), addresses externalizing behavioral symptomatology almost exclusively and, therefore, would not be sensitive to attention problems. It contains items such as "does the child sit still?" or "does the child disrupt games?" The SCRS indicates specific areas of treatment and includes an area where specific examples of impulsive behaviors can be written out.

10.2.1.5. Child Behavior Checklist

The Child Behavior Checklist[26] (CBCL) is a multidimensional (broad-based) parent questionnaire applicable to ages 4 to 16 years. Although it is a lengthy checklist (138 items), three scales of social competence (consisting of 20 items) and nine scales dealing with specific childhood diagnostic categories (118 items) are derived (e.g., depression, hyperactivity, somatic complaints). The hyperactivity scale is most useful in assessment of attention problems; however, the large item pool coupled with the many symptom scales, allows for better differentiation of ADD and other behavior problems. Scoring is rather cumbersome, but a computer format is available. (The CBCL is discussed below in more detail).

10.2.1.6. Revised Behavioral Problems Checklist

The Revised Behavioral Problems Checklist[27] (R-BPC) is another multidimensional scale that enables assessment of both externalizing and internalizing behavioral domains for grades K to 12 (the R-BPC is reviewed in more detail in Section 10.3.4.).

10.2.1.7. Aggregate Neurobehavioral Student Health and Education Review

The Aggregate Neurobehavioral Student Health and Education Review[28–30] (ANSER) is applicable to three age levels: 4 to 6 years, 6 to 11 years, and 12+ years of age. In addition, there is also a self-administered form, applicable from age 9 years and older. The ANSER contains more than 270 questions plus additional items that require written responses. This instrument yields a wealth of information, e.g., specific skills and abilities, interests, and associated strengths. The ANSER also provides an evaluation of attention that is more detailed than most questionnaires. Unfortunately, the excessive length, coupled with psychometric weaknesses regarding reliability, validity, and normative data,[28] detract from its potential usefulness. A brief form (20 items), the Abbreviated ANSER,[31] measures attention, strengths, activity, and behavior. The brevity of the instrument is clinically attractive, but the benefit may be offset by the small item pool that limits the amount of information that can be obtained.

10.2.1.8. Home Situations Questionnaire

The Home Situations Questionnaire[12] (HSQ) contains 16 items that depict home and public situations where parents observe and manage children's behaviors (e.g., "playing alone," "watching TV," or "when asked to do school homework"). The HSQ was designed to evaluate *where* children and adolescents may be exhibiting their problem behaviors versus what *type* of problems they may be having.[32] Two summary scores are provided: (1) Number of Problem Situations, which indicates situational diversity (scored yes/no), and (2) a Mean Severity Score for all situations rated as problematic (range 1—mild—to 9—severe).

Delineation of situations in which problem behaviors occur is important because hyperactive children generally have fewer problems while playing alone or when the father is at home. However, these children have significant difficulties when their parents are on the phone, when they are asked to do chores, or when company is visiting the home.[32]

The HSQ yields four factors[32]: nonfamily transaction, task performance, custodial transaction, and isolate play. Strengths of the HSQ include the ability to evaluate specific aspects of problems versus global impressions that are obtained over situations. Moreover, the HSQ is sensitive to interventions and can identify deviance from normality.

Normative data are available for children from aged 4 to 18 years.[32,33] The mean number of problem settings for boys is 3.1 to 4.1 (depending on age), whereas the mean number of problem settings for girls ranges from 2.2 to 3.4 (the 6- to 8-year-old age range has the highest number, regardless of gender). The mean severity score for boys ranges from 1.7 to 2.0; for girls the range is 1.3 to 1.6.

There also is a revised Home Situations Questionnaire (HSQ-R).[32,34] This revision, applicable for ages 6 to 12 years, contains 14 items that are designed to assess specific problems with attention and concentration across a variety of home and public situations. It is recommended that the original HSQ be used where assessment of general behavior problems (e.g., oppositional or aggressive behavior) is the primary focus; the HSQ-R version should be employed when a more refined measure of attention deficits is needed.[32]

10.2.1.9. Children's Attention and Adjustment Survey

The Children's Attention and Adjustment Survey[35] (CAAS) is a behavioral rating scale for children aged 5 to 13 years, designed specifically to assess behavior problems related to hyperactivity. The survey requires approximately 5 min to complete and is applicable to both home (Home Form) and school (School Form). Each scale contains 31 items, such as "talks too much," "gets excited easily," or "inattentive, distractible." These items are scored on a four-point "how characteristic?" scale: 1 = "not at all," 2 = "a little," 3 = "quite a bit," and 4 = "very much."

There are several features of the CAAS that make it attractive for office use. The survey provides four scales: (1) inattentiveness, (2) impulsivity, (3) hyperactivity, and (4) conduct problems/aggressiveness. It is compatible with the DSM-III-R, and scoring is easy, with scales being computed in a two-page, hand-scorable booklet.

The CAAS, normed on 4000 children in grades K to 5, is based on an *interactive systems model*. This model considers home factors, specific symptoms, school behaviors, and physician orientation toward the diagnosis and treatment of a child referred for suspected ADHD.[35] Moreover, the authors go to great lengths to preserve the attention deficit with and without hyperactivity (ADHD, ADDWO) distinction. This has implications in terms of intervention. Comparison of both forms also is very helpful. However, in a sample of 178 children, correlations between parent and teacher ratings were $r = 0.34$ for inattention, $r = 0.30$ for ADHD, $r = 0.29$ for ADD, $r = 0.26$ for hyperactivity, $r = 0.10$ for conduct problems, and $r = 0.04$ for impulsivity.[35] The low correlations in the last two categories may reflect differences in item content between the Home and School Forms.[35]

A profile sheet is provided that affords visual comparison of where the major problems are, namely, inattention, impulsivity, hyperactivity, or conduct problems (or some combination).

Standard scores (ranging from 75 to 145), percentiles, stanines, and cut-off scores are provided. For example, in regard to cut-off scores on the School Form, a score ≥ 10 is significant for inattention, ≥ 5 for impulsivity, ≥ 8 for hyperactivity, and ≥ 16 for conduct problems. Use of these cut-off scores yields a 74% to 77% sensitivity (true positives based on physician diagnosis) but a 12% to 25% rate of false positives. The authors suggest that use of these cut-off scores in conjunction with additional data such as age of onset and pervasiveness enhances diagnostic accuracy.

In summary, the CAAS is useful in office practice, and it is a good, narrow-band *screening* instrument.

10.2.1.10. Attention-Deficit Disorders Evaluation Scale

The Attention-Deficit Disorders Evaluation Scale[36] (ADDES) is a relatively new scale, standardized on a total of almost 4900 children. Considerable attention was given to national representation of the normative sample, and reliability values are excellent. The Home Version Rating Scale contains 46 items, rated on a five-point scale: 0 = "does not engage in the behavior" to 4 = "one to several times per hour." Examples include, "needs oral questions and directions repeated frequently," "grabs things from others," and "makes excessive noise." Three types of scores are obtained: (1) raw scores for individual items, (2) subscale standard scores (0–20), and (3) percentile scores (see Figure 10.1).

Items from the ADDES group fall into three subscales: inattentive, impulsive, and hyperactive. The kit includes a 167-page intervention manual that contains the goals, objectives, and interventions for behaviors on the scale. Recommendations are phrased to fit nicely into Individual Educational Plans (IEPs) for children with ADHD. For example, for item 12, "has difficulty concentrating," a total of 36 interventions is provided. A computerized "Quick Score" program is available. The ADDES takes 12 to 15 min to complete.

The large normative sample, focus on the three main aspects of ADHD, and provision for interventions are attractive features of the ADDES. Unfortunately, at this time, there are little scientific research data

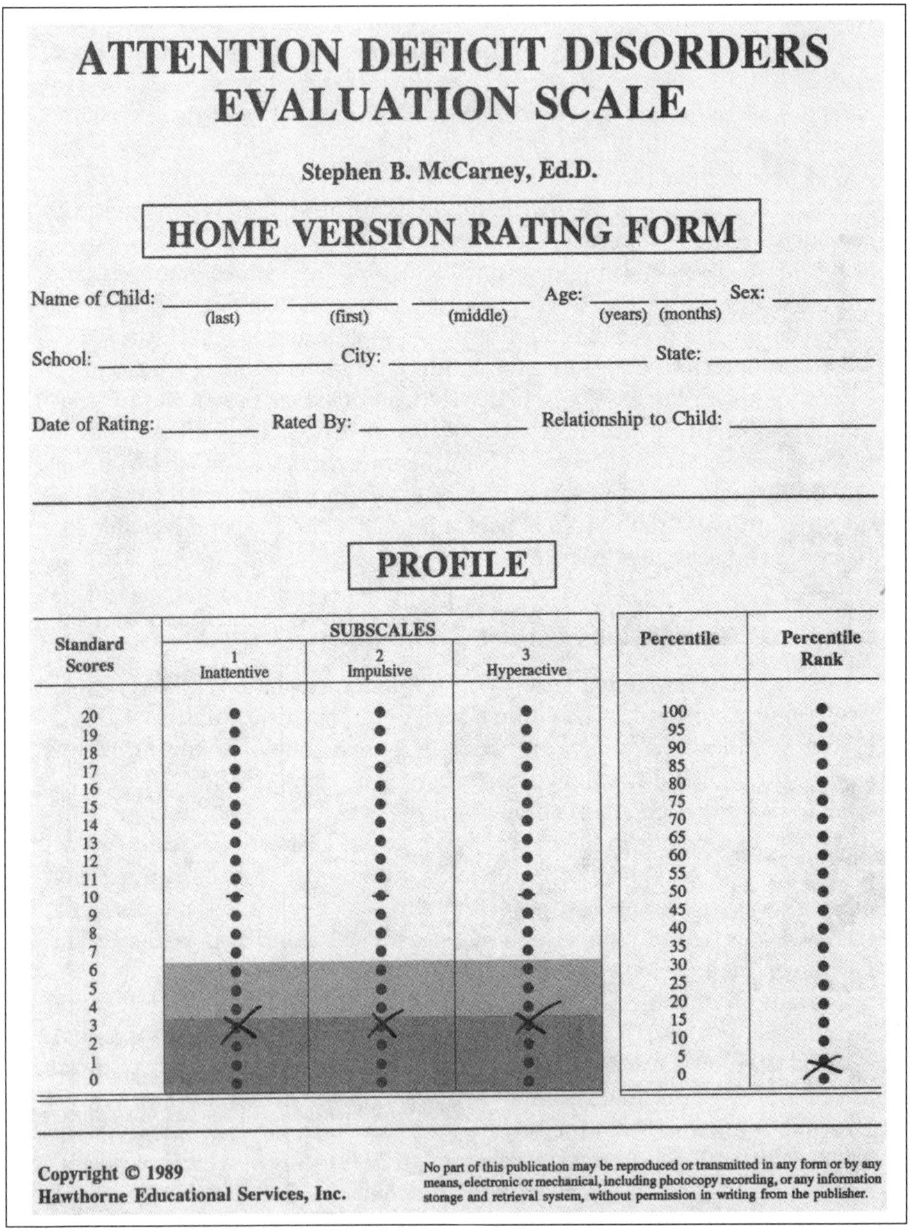

ATTENTION DEFICIT DISORDERS EVALUATION SCALE

Stephen B. McCarney, Ed.D.

HOME VERSION RATING FORM

Name of Child: ________ (last) ________ (first) ________ (middle) Age: _____ (years) _____ (months) Sex: ________

School: ________ City: ________ State: ________

Date of Rating: ________ Rated By: ________ Relationship to Child: ________

PROFILE

Standard Scores	SUBSCALES 1 Inattentive	2 Impulsive	3 Hyperactive	Percentile	Percentile Rank
20				100	
19				95	
18				90	
17				85	
16				80	
15				75	
14				70	
13				65	
12				60	
11				55	
10				50	
9				45	
8				40	
7				35	
6				30	
5				25	
4				20	
3				15	
2				10	
1				5	
0				0	

FIGURE 10.1. Attention Deficit Disorders Evaluation Scale (ADDES). (Copyright 1989, Hawthorne Educational Services. Reprinted with permission.)

available on the scale. The item content of the ADDES is similar to other scales, and there are a relatively large number of items. Pending additional research, the scale may be quite useful for the practitioner.

10.2.1.11. Summary

It is recommended that parent report measures be used in the evaluation of problems in attention and concentration. The Conners Parent Rating Scale (CPRS) is the traditional mainstay, but it tends to be narrow-band or unidimensional and encounters the risk of missing other problem areas that may mimic ADD. Although unidimensional assessments may not be useful for diagnosis per se, they are very effective in serial assessment or evaluation of treatment effects. Multidimensional questionnaires such as the CBCL are lengthy, yet they allow for more thorough evaluation of non-ADD behavioral dimensions. Clinicians will need to determine what is feasible for their individual practices, but at minimum, the CPRS and the HSQ (or Children's Attention and Adjustment Survey or Attention-Deficit Disorders Evaluation Scale) are recommended for routine use to establish baselines and evaluate treatment effects. Moreover, when disagreements between informants are found (e.g., between parents or between parents and teacher), these should not cause the clinician to dismiss the veracity of the informant's report. Discrepancies often provide information that is clinically valuable.

10.2.2. Teacher Rating Scales

Teachers often are regarded as being more reliable and sensitive to the nuances of behavior than are parents. Moreover, teachers are familiar with how the "typical" child should behave in the school setting. Conversely, teachers' ratings are prone to halo and practice effects. In fact, as mentioned previously, it has been suggested that teachers complete two questionnaires as baseline measures, because ratings generally improve between the first and second administration (regardless of whether or not intervention has been instituted).

Several parent questionnaires outlined in Table 10.1 have corresponding teacher forms. These include the Conners Teacher Rating Scales (four versions),[16–19] the Children's Behavior Checklist-Teacher Report Form,[8,26] SNAP-R,[24] CLAM,[21] ANSER,[29–31] Revised Behavior Problem Checklist,[27] the YCI,[23] Children's Attention and Adjustment Survey,[35] and the ADDES.[36] Comments regarding the parent versions of these questionnaires also are germane to the teacher forms. Obviously, there is a distinct advantage in having both the parent and teacher(s) complete similar questionnaires (see Table 10.2). Several of these teacher rating scales are discussed below.

10.2.2.1. Conners Teacher Rating Scale

The original Conners Teacher Rating Scale[16] (TRS) consists of 39 items, whereas the revised version contains only 28 items.[19] There is also a ten-item Conners Abbreviated Teacher Questionnaire (Hyperactivity Index), which appears to be sensitive to both hyperactivity and conduct disorders. This feature may cause confusion by diagnostically combining a mixed group of hyperactive/conduct-disordered patients.[37] Depending on the CTRS version that is employed (there are four versions in use),[32] several scales are derived: (1) conduct problem, (2) hyperactivity, (3) inattentive–passive, (4) emotional–overindulgent, (5) anxious–passive, and (6) asocial. The first three are found with the revised (28-item) CTRS. Agreement between the Parent and Teacher Conners ranges from $r = 0.33$ to $r = 0.45$.[16] The CTRS appears most useful as a screen for conduct problems and hyperactivity, and the best normative data are for ages 4 to 12 years.[38]

10.2.2.2. IOWA Conners Teacher Rating Scale

The IOWA Conners Teacher Rating Scale[22] (Inattention, Overactivity, With Aggression) contains ten items derived from the original CTRS (five pertaining to conduct problems and five measuring hyperactivity). This instrument, scored on a four-point scale, yields inattention/overactivity and aggression factors.[39] Sample items include "fidgeting," "inattentive," and "acts smart." The primary utility of the scale is to identify children who are hyperactive, aggressive, or both.[32] Actually, there is a parent version available, but its use has been limited, and it therefore remains obscure.

10.2.2.3. ADD-H Comprehensive Teacher Rating Scale

The ADD-H Comprehensive Teacher Rating Scale[40,41] (ACTeRS) has both clinical and research applications. Attention, Hyperactivity, Social Skills, and Oppositional realms are measured, with the use of 24 items on a scale of 1 to 5. Advantages of the ACTeRS include: (1) availability of norms based on gender, (2) sensitivity to the effects of psychopharmacological

TABLE 10.2. Teacher Rating Scales

Scale	Ages/grades	Number of items	Type of assessment	Teacher form available	Publisher
Conners Teachers Rating Scale (CTRS)	3–17 years	28	Narrow-band	Y	MultiHealth Systems
IOWA Conners Teacher Rating Scale	Grade 1–5	10	Narrow-band	N	Authors
ADD-H Comprehensive Teacher Rating Scale (ACTeRS)	5–12 years	24	Narrow-band	N	MetriTech
Child Attention Problems (CAP)	6–16 years	12	Narrow-band	N	Author
School Situations Questionnaire (SSQ)	4–11 years	12	Narrow-band	Y	Author
Swanson, Nolan, and Pelham Rating Scale (SNAP)	6–11 years	23	Narrow-band	Y	Author
Child Behavior Checklist-Teacher Report Form (CBCL-TRF)	6–16 years	126	Broad-band	Y	University of Vermont
Revised Behavioral Problems Checklist (R-BPC)	5–17 years	89	Broad-band	Y	Author
Aggregate Neurobehavioral Student Health and Education Review (ANSER)	4–6 years/6–11 years/12+ years	270	Broad-band	Y	Educators Publishing Service
Children's Attention and Adjustment Survey (CAAS)	5–13 years K–5	31	Narrow-band	Y	American Guidance Service
Attention Deficit Disorders Evaluation Scale (ADDES)	4–18 years	60	Narrow-band	Y	Hawthorne Educational Services

intervention, (3) assessment of several different areas of function, and (4) a profile sheet to which scores from the rating form can be transferred and displayed graphically. This last feature is very helpful in enhancing discussions with parents. Negative aspects include increased potential for rater bias effects because of the identification of factors on the rating sheet, the need for more data on reliability and validity, and the fact that there is no guidance in scoring, other than ranking the two extreme scores. Therefore, the midpoint score may be interpreted incorrectly as "average"[11,37] (see Figure 10.2). Scores below the tenth percentile are interpreted as being indicative of ADD, whereas those between the tenth and 25th percentiles suggest some deficit. This scale seems helpful in differentiating ADD children with and without hyperactivity; however, the authors' claim that the ACTeRS differentiates ADD from learning disabilities is questionable.

10.2.2.4. Edelbrock Child Attention/Activity Profile

The 12-item Edelbrock Child Attention/Activity Profile[42] (CAP) was derived from selected items of the Child Behavior Checklist Teacher Report form (in particular, items that tap inattention and overactivity). This instrument was specifically developed to assess effects of stimulant medication. The CAP contains the best discriminators of attention and activity that are found in the CBCL teacher form. Items are scored 0 ("not true") to 2 ("very or often true"). The upper limit of the normal range is 15 for boys and 11 for girls.[32] Further evaluation and wider application of this scale appear necessary.

10.2.2.5. School Situations Questionnaire

The School Situations Questionnaire[4,32] (SSQ) is the teacher counterpart of the Home Situations Questionnaire (HSQ). It contains 12 items that depict specific school and classroom situations in which children may display behavioral problems (e.g., "at recess," "doing in-seat work"). Factor analysis[33] of the SSQ has produced three areas of measurement: unsupervised settings, task performance, and special events. As with the HSQ, scores reflecting the number of problem situations and mean severity scores are produced. Social interaction, focused attention, and behavior in novel activities/situations are assessed.

The SSQ provides a situational profile that is useful in the development of behavioral interventions in the classroom. As with the HSQ, the School Situations Questionnaire confounds ratings of conduct problems with those of ADHD.[32] The mean number of problem sittings for boys ranges from 2.4 to 2.8; for girls the range is 1.0 to 1.3. The mean severity rating for boys is 1.5 to 1.9 and for girls, 0.8.[33]

There also is a revised School Situations Questionnaire[34] (SSQ-R), which contains eight items. The SSQ-R is designed specifically to assess attention and concentration problems. Whereas the mean number of problem settings is similar for males and females, mean severity ratings are somewhat higher (2.99–3.81 for girls, and 3.14–4.82 for boys).[32]

Additional teacher checklists, which correspond to the parent checklists discussed previously, are found in Table 10.2.

10.2.2.6. Summary

Teacher report measures are a critical component in the evaluation of academic problems. Clinicians are required to select unidimensional (narrow-band) and multidimensional (broad-band) assessments, based on individual circumstances; however, teacher reports are *essential* in the overall work-up. Difficulty in selection is compounded further because longer questionnaires yield more information, but there is a corresponding reluctance by some teachers to complete these longer checklists. As a baseline, administration of checklists such as the Conners Teacher Rating Scale (CTRS; 28 item) or the ADD-H Comprehensive Teacher Rating Scale (ACTeRS), supplemented by the School Situations Questionnaire (SSQ), is recommended. This protocol would enable evaluation of more stable, problem behaviors (which occur in any setting) as well as specific situations that result in problem behaviors.

Both parent and teacher rating scales should be used in the evaluation of school problems that are suggestive of ADD. However, a recent meta-analysis of parent–teacher agreement in symptom reporting indicated a mean agreement of $r = 0.20$.[43] Conversely, in clinical situations where a parent report is positive for attention problems, it is highly likely that the teacher report will also be positive.[44] Therefore, diagnosis based on both measures enhances certainty.[45]

10.3. MULTIDIMENSIONAL RATING SCALES

Several rating scales offer a more "broad-band" or multidimensional assessment. As indicated earlier, this type of assessment instrument allows for differentiation of problems in attention and concentration from other problems such as anxiety, depression, or oppositional behavior. Several of the most frequently used multidimensional rating scales are found in Table 10.3.

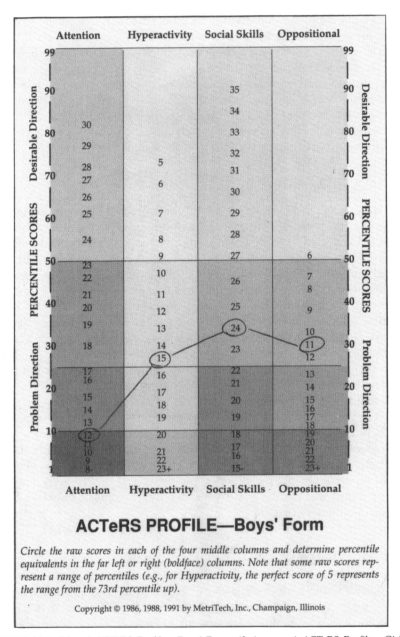

ACTeRS PROFILE—Boys' Form

Circle the raw scores in each of the four middle columns and determine percentile equivalents in the far left or right (boldface) columns. Note that some raw scores represent a range of percentiles (e.g., for Hyperactivity, the perfect score of 5 represents the range from the 73rd percentile up).

Copyright © 1986, 1988, 1991 by MetriTech, Inc., Champaign, Illinois

FIGURE 10.2. (above) ACTeRS Profile—Boys' Form. (facing page) ACTeRS Profile—Girls' Form. (ACTeRS Profile Form is copyright 1986, 1988, and 1991 by MetriTech, Inc., Champaign, IL. Reproduced by permission of the copyright holder.)

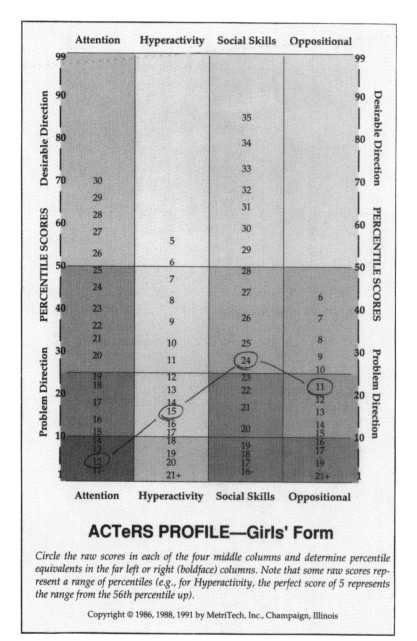

ACTeRS PROFILE—Girls' Form

Circle the raw scores in each of the four middle columns and determine percentile equivalents in the far left or right (boldface) columns. Note that some raw scores represent a range of percentiles (e.g., for Hyperactivity, the perfect score of 5 represents the range from the 56th percentile up).

FIGURE 10.2. (*Continued*)

TABLE 10.3. Multidimensional Rating Scales

Scale	Age	Number of items	Areas assessed	Parent/teacher form	Publisher
Child Behavior Checklist (CBCL)	4–18	126–138	Internalizing, Externalizing, Other	P/T	University of Vermont
Personality Inventory for Children (PIC)	6–16	131–600 (four versions)	Discipline/self-control Social Internalization Cognitive	P	Western Psychological Services
Louisville Behavior Checklist (LBC)	4–6/7–12/13–17	164	19 scales (aggression, hyperactivity, fear, etc. + severity)	P	Western Psychological Services
Revised Behavior Problem Checklist (R-BPC)	5–17 (K–12)	89	Conduct problems Socialized aggression Attention problems Immaturity Anxiety–withdrawal Psychotic behavior Motor tension—excess	P/T	Author
Behavior Assessment System for Children (BASC)	4–18	108–148 (teacher) 126–138 (parent)	DSM-III-R IDEA categories Adaptive (positive) Behavior Clinical (negative) Behavior	P/T/S	American Guidance Service
Devereux Behavior Rating Scales	5–12 13–18	135–136	Full range of pathology DSMIII-R/DSM IV	P/T	The Psychological Corp.

10.3.1. Child Behavior Checklist

The Child Behavior Checklist[46] (CBCL) often is considered the "gold standard" in the assessment of children's behavior problems.[47] The instrument was designed to provide standardized descriptions of behavior for children ages 4 to 18 years. Earlier versions[26] were applicable from ages 4 to 16 years (CBCL/4–16); the 1991 profiles still are comparable to earlier forms, but they focus more specifically on syndromes common to both sexes and different age ranges. There have been only minimal changes in the actual items. The CBCL is designed to be completed by the parent (a fifth-grade reading level is necessary), the goal being to obtain a profile of the child's behavior from the parent's perspective. The instrument, which requires approximately 15 to 20 min to complete, can be hand or computer scored. As noted previously, the CBCL consists of 138 items, 20 of which are social-competence items. These group into three categories: (1) activities (sports, hobbies, games), (2) social (organizations, jobs, chores), and (3) school (special class, repeated a grade). These behaviors are listed by the parent and are then rated on a four-point scale ("don't know," "less than average," "average," or "more than average"), both for time spent in the activity or how well the child performs in the particular activity. A total competence score is derived, with a T-score <37 falling into the clinical range, and a score of 37 to 40 being in the borderline clinical range.

The remaining 118 items comprise the Behavior Problems Scales. Parents are asked to rate a behavior such as "acts before thinking," "moody," or "stubborn" as 0 (not true), 1 (somewhat/sometimes true), or 2 (very true/often true). The CBCL yields eight problem scales (syndromes) at each age (one additional scale, "sex problems," is applicable only to ages 4 to 5 and 6 to 11 years). These scales are normed by age and gender and group into: (1) *Internalizing Behaviors* (withdrawn, somatic complaints, anxious/depressed), (2) *Externalizing Behaviors* (delinquent, aggressive), and (3) *Neither Internalizing Nor Externalizing Behaviors* (social problems, thought problems, attention problems, and sex problems). Behaviors falling in the internalizing group reflect overcontrol, such as being fearful or inhibited, whereas those in the externalizing grouping are uncontrolled, i.e., aggressive or antisocial. Scores falling above the 90th percentile (T-score >70) are of clinical significance. Sample items include "acts too young for his/her age," "daydreams or gets lost in his/her thoughts," and "gets in many fights."[46]

Regardless of sex/age grouping, the highest interparent agreement on the competence scale was for the school grouping ($r = 0.87$); the lowest was for activities ($r = 0.59$). On the problem scales, the highest interparent agreement was for social problems ($r = 0.73$), attention problems ($r =$

0.79), delinquent behavior ($r = 0.78$), and aggressive behavior ($r = 0.79$). The lowest scores were for somatic ($r = 0.52$), thought ($r = 0.45$), and sex problems ($r = 0.52$).[46]

As indicated earlier, there is a teacher report form (for ages 6–18) consisting of 126 items. An adaptive functions profile replaces the social competence profile and includes the child's work habits and level of academic performance. Factors include unpopular, inattentive, nervous–overactive, as well as anxious, social withdrawal, self-destructive, obsessive–compulsive, and aggressive. A self-rated Youth Self-Report Form (CBCL-YSR), applicable for ages 11 to 18 years, also is available. Worded in the first person, the CBCL-YSR contains two separate scales: (1) Competence (activities and social) and (2) Behavior Problems (which include broadband and narrow-band factors). However, reliability and validity of self-report instruments in children and adolescents are not as psychometrically sound as rating scales completed by parents or teachers.[32]

In addition to detecting psychoeducational problems, the CBCL is useful in screening for psychopathology in primary-care pediatric settings.[48] Physicians should be cautious in using the CBCL with chronically ill patients[47] because of limited sensitivity in picking up mild problems. It should be noted that in general pediatric populations physicians identify more children with psychosocial problems than does the CBCL.[49] Nonetheless, in most cases Child Behavior Checklist T-scores were ≥50 in the children identified by the physician but not the test instrument, suggesting that diagnostic thresholds of the CBCL might be too high. Stability of internalizing scales is lower than that of externalizing scales; declines in six of eight behavior problem scales over a 4-month period have also been reported, even when no intervention was provided. This should be a consideration in any type of treatment program. Some items are scored on more than one narrow-band scale, and this inflates intercorrelations between scales and limits the discriminant validity of the items.[50] The inattention scale also reportedly differentiates ADD with and without hyperactivity.[51] The CBCL subscales correlate well with the Conners scales and the Revised Behavior Problem Checklist.

10.3.2. Personality Inventory for Children

The Personality Inventory for Children[52–54] (PIC) is not a child behavior rating scale per se but rather an inventory of personality characteristics in children. It is scored "true/false" and designed to be completed by a parent (sixth- to seventh-grade reading level is necessary). The applicable age range is 6 to 16 years. In design the 600-item PIC is similar to the

Minnesota Multiphasic Personality Inventory (MMPI) in that there are both validity scales and clinical scales. The three validity scales include: (1) a lie scale (denial of commonly occurring behavioral problems), (2) an F or frequency scale (contains items infrequently endorsed in the normative sample and that reflect deviancy or a random test-taking approach), and (3) a defensiveness scale (measures defensiveness in the parent). The 12 clinical scales are: (1) achievement, (2) intellectual screening, (3) a developmental scale (physical/verbal ability), (4) somatic concern, (5) hyperactivity, (6) social skills, (7) depression, (8) family relations, (9) delinquency, (10) withdrawal, (11) anxiety, and (12) psychosis.

Not all 600 items are necessary to generate a profile; 420-, 280-, or 131-item sets can be administered, although the number of useful critical items, clinical scales, or factor scales decreases accordingly. The first section of 131 items allows scoring of four scales and the Lie scale; completion of the first 280 items permits these factors to be scored as well as 12 abbreviated clinical scales and a general adjustment scale. The four factors include: (1) undisciplined/poor self-control, (2) social incompetence, (3) internalization/somatic symptoms, and (4) cognitive development. Generally, the higher the T-score on a given scale, the greater the likelihood of problems; however, the range of clinical significance varies by scale. For example, a T-score of >59 is significant for the hyperactivity scale, but a score of >69 is significant for social skills. Interparental agreement ranges from 0.57 to 0.69. The PIC is useful in differentiating hyperactive, learning-disabled, and normal children as well as learning-disabled versus behaviorally disordered students.[54,55] Sample items include "has few or no friends," "can't sit still," "has problems learning in school," and "doesn't finish things."[52,54] It is recommended that the 280- or 131-item versions be used in clinical practice because these afford a balance between length of time needed to complete the task and the amount of information obtained. The longer version can require 1 to 2 hr for a parent to complete. The PIC can be hand or computer scored.

10.3.3. Louisville Behavior Checklist

The Louisville Behavior Checklist[56] (LBC) contains three forms: 4 to 6 years, 7 to 12, and 13 to 17 years. Each form contains 164 "true–false" items that are completed by the child's caretaker. Each form contains 13 to 19 scales, depending upon the child's age. Eleven factors are assessed, and these include aggression, inhibition, infantile aggression, antisocial behavior, social withdrawal, hyperactivity, sensitivity, fear, learning disability, and immaturity. Four factors are particularly pertinent in regard to problems in school performance: (1) learning disability, (2) hyperactivity, (3) academic disability, and (4) immaturity. Parents need a tenth-grade reading level to complete this true–false checklist, which requires 20 to 30 min for administration; scoring requires 10 min. Use is not widespread at present, and the normative sample is relatively small. However, it can be a useful screen in primary care.

10.3.4. Behavior Problem Checklist/Revised Behavior Problem Checklist

The Behavior Problem Checklist[27,57,58] (BPC) is a frequently used checklist completed by parents, teachers, or other informants for children aged 5 to 13 years. Four factors are produced: (1) conduct problems, (2) personality problems, (3) inadequate–immature, and (4) socialized delinquency. The 55 items contained in the BPC are scaled 0 (does not constitute a problem), 1 (mild problem), and 2 (severe problem); raw scores are again converted into T-scores ($M = 50$, $SD = 10$). The newer Revised Behavior Problem Checklist contains 89 items, and normative data are available for parent and teacher ratings for children from grades K through 12 (ages 5–17 years). Interparent agreement ranges between $r = 0.55$ and 0.93. On the RBPC, six factors are assessed: (1) conduct disorder, (2) socialized aggression, (3) attention problems–immaturity, (4) anxiety–withdrawal, (5) psychotic behavior, and (6) motor tension excess. Administration time is 15 to 20 min. The RBPC is reported to differentiate ADD children with and without hyperactivity.

10.3.5. Behavior Assessment System for Children

The Behavior Assessment System for Children[59] (BASC) is a new, "multi-method" approach to evaluating both the behavior and self-perceptions of children aged 4 to 18 years. It is multimethod in that the BASC contains five components: (1) a self-report scale (SRP) (in which the child describes his/her concerns and self-perceptions), (2) a teacher rating scale (TRS), (3) parent rating scales (PRS), (4) a structured developmental history, and (5) a form to record directly observed classroom behavior. The system also is "multidimensional" in that it measures numerous aspects of behavior, including positive (adaptive) as well as negative (clinical) dimensions. The focus of the BASC is more on diagnosis than screening.

The BASC is compatible with the DSM-III-R as well as categories of problems addressed by the Individuals with Disabilities Education Act

(IDEA). Another attractive feature, similar to that found with the Wechsler Individual Achievement Test (Chapter 8), is that information from multiple sources can be compared using instruments that are conormed.

10.3.5.1. BASC Teacher Rating Scales

The Teacher Rating Scales (TRS) has three forms: (1) preschool (ages 4–5 years), (2) child (ages 6–11), and (3) adolescent (12–18 years). The forms contain from 108 to 148 descriptors of behaviors (e.g., "worries," "says 'nobody likes me,'" "blames others"), which are rated on a four-point scale of frequency from "never" to "almost always." The TRS requires 10 to 20 min to complete. Externalizing Problems (aggression, hyperactivity, conduct problems), Internalizing Problems (anxiety, depression, somatization), School Problems (attention, learning), and Adaptive Skills (adaptibility, leadership, social skills, study skills) are measured. An "F" (fake bad) index provides a validity check, designed to detect a negative response set on the part of the teacher.

10.3.5.2. BASC Parent Rating Scales

Similar to the TRS, the Parent Rating Scales (PRS) has three forms containing from 126 to 138 items. It utilizes the same four-choice response format (e.g., "is overly active," "teases others," "is sad"). The same clinical problems and adaptive behavior domains are addressed as on the teacher form, with the exception of the School Problems Composite or the Learning Problems and Study Skills scales. An "F" index is included.

10.3.5.3. BASC Self-Report of Personality

The Self-Report of Personality (SRP) is a true/false personality inventory available for two age levels: child (8–11 years) and adolescent (12–18 years). The SRP requires 30 min to complete, and several composite scores are produced: (1) School Maladjustment, (2) Clinical Maladjustment, (3) Personal Adjustment, and (4) an overall composite score, the Emotional Symptoms Index. The child level has a total of 12 scales, the adolescent level 14 scales.

In addition, there also are a Structured Developmental History (which can be completed by the clinician during an interview or may be completed as a questionnaire by the parent) and a Student Observation System (a form for directly recording the classroom behavior of a child). The observation system allows recording of positive and negative behaviors.

Review of the BASC indicates mediocre correlations between parent and teacher forms ($r = 0.25$ for Atypicality scales, $r = 0.34$ for the Depression parent and teacher scales).[59] Similar findings were noted between the self-report and parent and teacher rating scales (self-report depression correlates 0.20 with teacher-rated depression and 0.26 with parent-rated depression).

The BASC scales yield a mean T-score of 50 and a SD of 10; scores above 70 are considered significantly high, whereas those less than 30 are considered to be significantly low. Scores in the 60 to 69 and 31 to 40 ranges are considered "at risk." The "average" T-score range is 41 to 59.

The mean BASC correlations with the CBCL-Teacher Report Form are in the $r = 0.45$ to 0.59 range for the child level (the highest correlation, incidentally, was for attention problems) and $r = 0.46$ to 0.59 at the adolescent level.[59] The BASC has considerable content overlap with the Revised Behavior Problem Checklist[58] in regard to externalizing and school problems. Although there is some overlap with the Conners Teachers Rating Scale (39-item version),[18] these two instruments clearly measure different behaviors.

The BASC has many attractive features; however, because the assessment system is so new, the scientific data that have been collected thus far are limited. Clinicians would find the BASC useful, and it allows far better delineation of behavioral problems than many other scales.

10.3.6. Devereux Behavior Rating Scales

The new Devereux Behavior Rating Scales[60] are available in two forms, *The Devereux School Form* and *The Devereux Clinical Form*. These forms are newly developed and restandardized versions of the Devereux Behavior Rating Scales, originally published in the mid-1960s. Each scale has two levels with separate sets of items that are appropriate for younger children (5–12 years) and adolescents (13–18 years). Separate norms for males and females were developed, using more than 3000 cases.

10.3.6.1. Devereux Clinical Form

The clinical form contains 135 to 136 items (depending on age) and requires 15 min for the caretaker to complete. Items are scored 1 (never) to 5 (very frequently), with the caretaker answering the question "During the past 4 weeks, how often did the child . . . ," "argue with adults," "have temper tantrums," "get easily distracted," etc. The clinical form can be completed by a relative/guardian or school personnel.

10.3.6.2. Devereux School Form

The school form consists of 40 items and requires 5 min to complete. This screening device is formatted in a manner similar to the clinical form (i.e., 1 = never to 5 = very frequently).

Items and directions are written at a sixth-grade level, and content validity of the revised scales is based primarily on DSM-III-R diagnostic criteria and federal regulations for defining "serious emotional disturbance" under PL 94-142.

A comparison of the Devereux School Form and the Child Behavior Checklist—Teacher Report Form[46] indicates that the CBCL-TRF has somewhat higher sensitivity than the Devereux but that the Devereux has higher specificity. Both scales correctly identified approximately 75% of the sample, and both were considered useful in the identification of seriously emotionally disturbed students.[61]

The Devereux scales will be useful for practitioners, particularly when the issue of serious emotional disturbance (SED) is raised. The scales have just become available, so there are few scientific studies available at this time that address the applicability of the instrument.

10.3.7. Conclusions

The primary-care physician typically is faced with a plethora of rating scales, many of which have not been included in this chapter. In addition, there are many peer-rating, self-rating, and observational techniques available. Nonetheless, adequate selection of narrow-band parent and teacher rating scales and multidimensional instruments can readily be made from the scales that have been outlined. It should be emphasized that the majority of these scales offer descriptions of behaviors and do not produce a true diagnosis per se (the Behavior Assessment System for Children— BASC—being an exception). Behavioral questionnaires should be used routinely as a component in the evaluation of problems in school performance and academic achievement.

REFERENCES

1. Eisert, D. C., Sturner, R. A., and Mabe, P. A., 1991, Questionnaires in behavioral pediatrics: Guidelines for selection and use, *J. Dev. Behav. Pediatr.* **12:**42–50.
2. Naglieri, J. A., and Flanagan, D. P., 1992, A psychometric review of behavior rating scales, *Comp. Ment. Health Care* **2:**225–239.

3. Sturner, R. A., Eisert, D. C., and Mabe, A., 1985, Questionnaire use in pediatric practice: Survey of practice, *Clin. Pediatr.* **24:**638–641.

4. Barkley, R. A., and Edelbrock, C., 1987, Assessing situational variation in children's problem behaviors: The home and school situations questionnaires, in: *Advances in Behavioral Assessment of Children and Families*, Volume 3 (R. J. Prinz, ed.), JAI Press, Greenwich, CT, pp. 157–176.

5. Eyberg, S., 1980, Eyberg Child Behavior Inventory, *J. Clin. Child Psychol.* **9:**22–28.

6. O'Leary, K. D., and Johnson, S. B., 1979, Psychological assessment, in: *Psychopathological Disorders of Childhood*, ed. 2 (H. C. Quay and J. S. Werry, eds.), John Wiley & Sons, New York.

7. Achenbach, T. M., and Edelbrock, C. S., 1979, The child behavior profile: II. Boys aged 12–16 and girls aged 6–11 and 12–16, *J. Consult. Clin. Psychol.* **47:**223–233.

8. Edelbrock, C., and Achenbach, T. A., 1984, The teacher version of the Child Behavior Profile: I. Boys aged 6–11, *J. Consult. Clin. Psychol.* **52:**207–217.

9. Sattler, J. M., 1988, *Assessment of Children*, ed. 3, Jerome M. Sattler, San Diego, CA.

10. Sleator, F. K., and Ullman, R. A., 1981, Can the physician diagnose hyperactivity in the office? *Pediatrics* **67:**13–17.

11. Blondis, T. A., Accardo, P. J., and Snow, J. H., 1989, Measures of attention deficit. Part I. Questionnaires, *Clin. Pediatr.* **28:**222–228.

12. Barkley, R. A., 1991, Diagnosis and assessment of attention deficit–hyperactivity disorder, *Comp. Ment. Health Care* **1:**27–43.

13. Barkley, R. A., 1981, *Hyperactive Children: A Handbook for Diagnosis and Treatment*, Guilford Press, New York, pp. 113–155.

14. Kelly, D. P., and Aylward, G. P., 1992, Attention deficits in school aged children and adolescents: Current issues and practice, *Pediatr. Clin. North Am.* **39:**487–512.

15. Zelko, F. A. J., 1991, Comparison of parent-completed behavior rating scales: Differentiating boys with ADD from psychiatric and normal controls, *J. Dev. Behav. Pediatr.* **12:** 31–37.

16. Conners, C. K., 1969, A teacher rating scale for use in drug studies with children, *Am. J. Psychiat.* **127:**884.

17. Conners, C. K., 1973, Rating scales for use in drug studies with children, *Psychopharmacol. Bull.* (special issue) **24-84.**

18. Conners, C. K., 1989, *Manual for Conners Rating Scales*, Multi-Health Systems, North Tonawanda, NY.

19. Goyette, C. H., Conners, C. K., and Ulrich, R. F., 1978, Normative data for Revised Conners Parent and Teacher Rating Scales, *J. Abnorm. Child Psychol.* **6:**221–236.

20. Ullmann, R. K., and Sleator, E. K., 1985, Attention deficit disorder children with or without hyperactivity, *Clin. Pediatr.* **24:**547–551.

21. Swanson, J. M., 1989, The Conners, Loney and Milich (CLAM) Questionnaire, unpublished manuscript, University of California, Irvine.

22. Atkins, M. S., and Milich, R., 1988, The IOWA Conners Rating Scale, in: *Dictionary of Behavioral Assessment Techniques* (A. S. Bellach and M. Herson, eds.), Pergamon Press, New York, pp. 273–275.

23. Shaywitz, S. E., Shaywitz, B. A., Schnell, C., and Towle, V. R., 1988, Concurrent and predictive validity of the Yale Children's Inventory: An instrument to assess children with attentional deficits and learning disabilities, *Pediatrics* **81:**562.

24. Pelham, W. E., Atkins, M. S., Murphy, H. A., and White, K. S., 1981, Operationalization and validation of attention deficit disorder, paper presented at annual meeting of the Association for Advancement of Behavioral Therapy, Toronto.

25. Kendall, P. C., and Wilcox, L. E., 1979, Self-control in children: Development of a rating scale, *J. Consult. Clin. Psychol.* **47:**1020–1029.
26. Achenbach, T. M., and Edelbrock, C., 1983, *Manual for the Child Behavior Checklist and Revised Child Behavior Profile*, Department of Psychiatry, University of Vermont, Burlington.
27. Quay, H. C., 1983, A dimensional approach to behavior disorder: The Revised Behavior Problem Checklist, *School Psychol. Rev.* **12:**244–249.
28. Harrington, R. G., 1985, Review of the ANSER System, in: *The Ninth Mental Measurements Yearbook* (J. V. Mitchell, ed.), Buros Institute of Mental Measurements, Lincoln, NE, pp. 77–78.
29. Levine, M. D., 1984, *The ANSER System (Aggregate Neurobehavioral Student Health and Educational Review)*, Educators Publishing Service, Cambridge, MA.
30. Levine, M. D., 1989, *The ANSER System: Interpreter's Guide*, Educators Publishing Service, Cambridge, MA.
31. Kelly, D. P., 1989, *Abbreviated ANSER Attention–Activity Questionnaire*, Southern Illinois University, Springfield.
32. Barkley, R. A., 1990, *Attention Deficit Hyperactivity Disorder. A Handbook for Diagnosis and Treatment*, Guilford Press, New York.
33. Breen, M. J., and Altepeter, T. S., 1991, Factor structures of the Home Situations Questionnaire and the School Situations Questionnaire, *J. Pediatr. Psychol.* **16:**59–67.
34. DuPaul, G. J., 1990, *The Home and School Situations Questionnaire—Revised: Normative data, reliability, and validity*, unpublished manuscript, University of Massachusetts Medical Center, Worcester.
35. Lambert, N., Hartsough, C., and Sandoval, J., 1990, *Manual for the Children's Attention and Adjustment Survey*, American Guidance Service, Circle Pines, MN.
36. McCarney, S. B., 1989, *Attention Deficit Disorders Evaluation Scale (ADDES)*, Hawthorne, Columbia, MO.
37. Barkley, R. A., 1988, Child behavior rating scales and checklists, in: *Assessment and Diagnosis in Child Psychopathology* (M. Rutter, H. Tuma, and I. Lann, eds.), Guilford Press, New York.
38. Trites, R. L., Blouin, A. G., and Laprade, K., 1982, Factor analysis of the Conners Teacher Rating Scale based on a large normative sample, *J. Consult. Clin. Psychol.* **50:**615–623.
39. Atkins, M. S., Pelham, W. E., and Licht, M. H., 1989, The differential validity of teacher ratings of inattention/overactivity and aggression, *J. Abnorm. Child Psychol.* **17:**423–435.
40. Ullmann, R. K., Sleator, E. K., and Sprague, R. L., 1984, A new rating scale for diagnosis and monitoring of ADD children, *Psychopharmacol. Bull.* **20:**160–165.
41. Ullman, R. K., Sleator, E. K., and Sprague, R. L., 1988, *Manual for the ADD-H Comprehensive Teacher's Rating Scale*, Metrotech, Champaign, IL.
42. Barkley, R. A., 1988, Attention, in: *Assessment Issues in Children Neuropsychology* (M. G. Tramontana and S. R. Hooper, eds.), Plenum Press, New York.
43. Achenbach, T. M., McConaughy, S. H., and Howell, C. T., 1987, Child/adolescent behavioral and emotional problems: Implications of cross-informant correlations for situational specificity, *Psychol. Bull.* **101:**213–232.
44. Biederman, J., Keenan, K., and Farone, S. V., 1990, Parent-based diagnosis of attention deficit disorder predicts a diagnosis based on teacher report, *J. Am. Acad. Child Adoles. Psychiat.* **29:**698–701.
45. Rutter, M., 1988, DSM III-R: A postscript, in: *Assessment and Diagnosis in Child Psychopathology* (M. Rutter, A. H. Tuma, and I. S. Lann, eds.), Guilford Press, New York, pp. 453–464.

46. Achenbach, T. M., 1991, *Manual for the Child Behavior Checklist/14–18 and 1991 Profile*, University of Vermont, Department of Psychiatry, Burlington.

47. Perrin, E. C., Stein, R. E., and Drotar, D., 1991, Cautions in using the Child Behavior Checklist: Observations based on research about children with a chronic illness, *J. Pediatr. Psychol.* **16:**411–421.

48. Costello, E. J., and Edelbrock, C. S., 1985, Detection of psychiatric disorders in pediatric primary care: A preliminary report, *J. Am. Acad. Child Psychiat.* **24:**771–774.

49. Horowitz, S. M., Leaf, P. J., Leventhal, J. M., Forsyth, B. W., and Speechley, K. N., 1991, Identifying sources of discrepancy between pediatrician's diagnoses and the Child Behavior Checklist, *Am. J. Dis. Child.* **145:**405.

50. MacMann, G. M., Barnett, D. W., Burd, S. A., et al., 1992, Construct validity of the Child Behavior Checklist: Effects of item overlap on second-order factor structure, *Psychol. Assess.* **4:**113–116.

51. Edelbrock, C., Costello, E. J., and Kessler, M. D., 1984, Empirical corroboration of attention deficit disorder, *J. Am. Acad. Child Psychiat.* **23:**285–290.

52. Lachar, D., and Gdowski, C. L., 1979, *Actuarial Assessment of Child and Adolescent Personality: An Interpretive Guide for the Personality Inventory for Children Profile*, Western Psychological Services, Los Angeles.

53. Lachar, D., Gdowski, C. L., and Snyder, D. K., 1984, External validation of the Personality Inventory for Children (PIC) profile and factor scales: parent, teacher and clinician ratings, *J. Consult. Clin. Psychol.* **52:**155–164.

54. Wirt, R. D., Lachar, D., Klinedinst, J. E., Seat, P. D., and Broen, W. E., 1984, *Personality Inventory for Children*, Western Psychological Services, Los Angeles.

55. Breen, M., and Barkley, R. A., 1983, The Personality Inventory for Children: Its clinical utility with hyperactive children, *J. Pediatr. Psychol.* **8:**359–366.

56. Miller, L. C., 1984, *Louisville Behavior Checklist*, Western Psychological Services, Los Angeles.

57. Quay, H. C., and Peterson, D. R., 1975, *Manual for the Behavior Problem Checklist*, unpublished manuscript, University of Miami.

58. Quay, H. C., and Peterson, D. R., 1987, *Manual for the Revised Behavior Problem Checklist*, University of Miami, Coral Gables, FL.

59. Reynolds, C. R., and Kamphaus, R. W., 1992, *BASC. Behavior Assessment System for Children Manual*, American Guidance Service, Circle Pines, MN.

60. Naglieri, J. A., LeBuffe, P. A., and Pfeiffer, S. A., 1993, *Devereux Behavior Rating Scales*, Psychological Corporation, San Antonio.

61. LeBuffe, P., Hess, R., Servis, L., and Waschbusch, D., 1992, *Identifying SED students: The Devereux Scales vs. the TRF*, paper presented at the 100th Annual Convention of the American Psychological Association, Washington, DC.

11 ✻ Visual–Motor/Visual–Perceptual Function

11.1. INTRODUCTION

Visual–motor and visual–perceptual dysfunction may have a significant, adverse influence on a child's school performance. Although visual–motor and visual–perceptual skills are highly interrelated, they also are distinct functions. A child with a visual–motor problem may not exhibit a visual–perceptual deficit; similarly, the reverse is also true (see Figure 11.1). If a child can draw rapidly (without excessive effort) but is unable to recognize that the reproduction differs markedly from the letter or shape being copied, there is a strong likelihood that an underlying perceptual deficit exists (Figure 11.1b). Conversely, if the child can recognize errors or discrepancies but, nonetheless, is unable to correct them, the probability of having a visual–motor problem is increased significantly (Figure 11.1c). A child who displays immature visual reproductions may be experiencing difficulty with the *integration* of perceptual and motor functions.[1,2]

Traditionally, visual–motor skills have been considered prerequisites for successful school performance, and these skills are heavily weighted in the assessment of school readiness. This concept originally evolved from an assumption that learning disabilities were primarily based on perceptual pathology. Research studies indicate that children with visual–motor deficits often have difficulty in early elementary grades with the acquisition of basic academic skills. However, these deficits are not as predictive of later reading difficulty as was once thought.[3] In fact, correlations between visual–motor test scores and reading skills generally are less than $r = 0.40$.[3] It should be noted that poor visual–motor and visual–perceptual skills may be associated with maturational delay, decreased intellectual abilities, neurological impairment, learning disabilities, attention-deficit disorders, or simply a lack of experience with visual or perceptual tasks.

Visual–motor performance conceptually involves four areas: (1) *stim-*

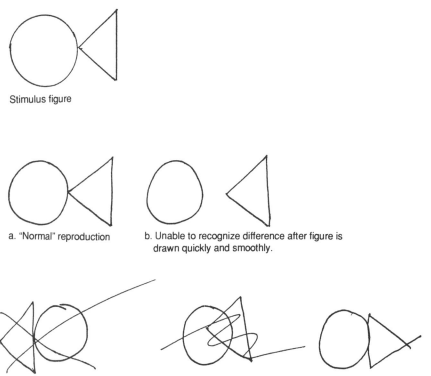

Stimulus figure

a. "Normal" reproduction

b. Unable to recognize difference after figure is drawn quickly and smoothly.

c. Can recognize mistake, but is unable to correct.

FIGURE 11.1. Visual–motor/visual–perceptual problems.

ulus reception and processing (looking at the letter or figure), (2) *sensory integration* (comparing the stimulus to information stored in long-term memory), (3) *effector activity* (making a decision to draw and then implementing the decision), and (4) *information feedback* (proprioceptive, kinesthetic, visual, verbal).[4] Deficits in any one of these areas, or in some combination, may produce functional problems.

It is recommended that health care providers conceptualize the potential areas of deficit as *misperception* (input), *execution problems* (fine motor output), or *integrative dysfunction* (processing). Clinicians should focus on the *process*, as well as the *product*, of a visual–motor task. Process factors include (1) handedness, (2) presence of motor overflow (mirroring of the other hand, tongue protrudes), (3) degree of impulsivity, (4) rotation of paper or stimulus materials, (5) difficulty with certain functions (diagonals, angles), (6) pencil pressure, (7) awareness of errors, (8) placement, and (9) erasures (and degree of improvement of production after erasure).[5] Children's reactions to their drawings are significant. Many children with visual–motor deficits are reluctant to draw, or they become very apologetic at the outset, frequently commenting that "I'm not good at drawing."

Visual–motor deficits also affect the quality of the child's human figure drawings, which in turn are assumed to be related to their general cognitive/intellectual development. In fact, many intelligence tests include a drawing component of some type (such as the McCarthy Scales of Children's Abilities or the Stanford–Binet Form L-M). Therefore, visual–motor and visual–perceptual deficits may produce an erroneous assumption that the child has compromised cognitive abilities. Figure drawings frequently are used in the evaluation of emotional functioning; however, visual–motor or visual–perceptual deficits again may result in incorrect interpretations.[6,7] Although discussion of these two areas of analysis of visual–motor function are beyond the purview of this chapter, the level of visual–motor function must be considered with any draw-a-person or other projective technique.

Generally, most tests used in the measurement of visual–motor function require that the child draw or copy various geometric designs onto a sheet of paper. Some tests, such as the Motor Free Visual Perception Test (MFVPT),[8] eliminate the motor component by having the child select items from a multiple-choice format. Test instruments may be grouped into three areas, those that (1) require reproduction of figures, (2) involve a memory component, and (3) evaluate visual perception only. These tests are summarized in Table 11.1.

11.2. TESTS THAT REQUIRE REPRODUCTION OF FIGURES

11.2.1. Bender Visual Motor Gestalt Test

The Bender-Gestalt Test (B-G) is by far the most frequently used paper-and-pencil task and is utilized by more than 90% of school psychologists. The test was developed from Gestalt psychology principles and originally was applied to adults to detect psychiatric and organic problems. The B-G requires that the child copy nine figures, each presented on a 4- × 6-inch card. The figures are copied on unlined $8\frac{1}{2}$- × 11-inch paper, the procedure taking approximately 5–10 min. Items to be reproduced include various dot configurations, circles, interrelated figures (circle and a rotated square, two hexagons), or intersecting lines.[1]

Multiple scoring systems are available; however, those developed by Koppitz[2,11] are used most frequently with children (the normative sample

TABLE 11.1. Tests That Measure Visual-Motor and Visual-Perceptual Function

Test	Age	Areas assessed			Publisher
		Visual motor	Visual perceptual	Visual memory	
Bender Visual Motor Gestalt Test (B-G)	5-0 to adult	X	X	–	American Orthopsychiatric Association
Modified Version of the Bender-Gestalt Test for Preschool Preschool and Primary School Children	4-6 to 8-5	X	X	–	Clinical Psychology Publishing Co.
Developmental Test of Visual Motor Integration (VMI)	2 to 15	X	X	–	The Psychological Corporation
Minnesota Percepto-Diagnostic Test (MPD)	5 to 14	X	X	–	Clinical Psychology Publishing Co.
Revised Visual Retention Test	7 to 14	X	–	X	The Psychological Corporation
Memory-for-Designs Test	7 to adult	X	–	X	The Psychological Corporation
Motor-Free Visual Perception Test	4 to 8-11	–	X	X	Western Psychological Services

consisted of 975 children). With this scoring scheme, 30 developmentally based types of errors are delineated. The errors include (1) rotations (45° or more), (2) distortions (destruction of the Gestalt; figure misshapen, disproportionate, or with parts substituted), (3) problems with integration (connection of parts, lines not crossed properly, shape is lost), or (4) perseveration (elements overproduced, excessive increase or continuation of parts) (see Figure 11.2). A developmental score, age equivalent, and percentile rank can be obtained for children from ages 5-0 to 10-11 years. Interjudge reliabilities cluster around $r = 0.90$; the mean correlation with intelligence test scores is $r = 0.48$.[2] Twelve emotional indicators have also been listed (e.g., small size, shading).

Most children produce a near-perfect performance by age 8 years; as a result, children 9 years of age or older who have mild to even moderate

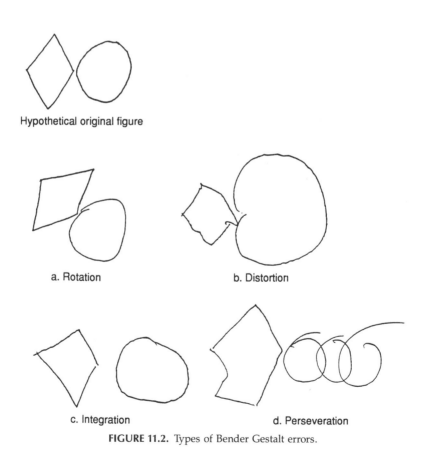

Hypothetical original figure

a. Rotation   b. Distortion

c. Integration   d. Perseveration

FIGURE 11.2. Types of Bender Gestalt errors.

visual–motor difficulties often are not identified. It must be emphasized that the B-G score is not a definitive indicator of brain damage, and it should *not* be used as such. However, it is an excellent "warm-up" task and is a very useful measure of visual–motor and visual–perceptual ability.

There are several variations in the administration procedure for the B-G. One variation is to request that all nine designs be placed on one page; this allows better evaluation of visual–organizational skills. A second alteration is to have the child draw as many designs as he/she can remember 5 min after completion of the B-G. Finally, a third variation is to reproduce as many designs as possible immediately after completion of the task.

11.2.2. Modified Version of the Bender-Gestalt Test for Preschool and Primary School Children[12]

The Modified Version of the Bender-Gestalt Test[12] was designed to measure the development of visual–motor integrative skills in children aged 4-6 to 8-5 (grades K through 2). The Modified B-G was normed on a sample of 994 children; interscorer reliability was $r = 0.95$. The test may be administered individually or in group settings.

This instrument incorporates six of the original B-G designs, eliminating three of the most difficult ones. A six-point scoring system is used, ranging from "0" (random drawing, scribbling) to "5" (perfect representation). Total scores therefore can range from 0 to 30. Percentile scores and T-scores are obtained for eight age groups. These standard and percentile scores also can be obtained for grades K, 1, and 2, based on either fall or spring testing.

The Modified B-G was "designed to provide a global measure of maturity of visual–motor integration skill" (p. 36).[12] It is this author's opinion, however, that the norms may be a bit too liberal, thereby lacking sensitivity in many cases; the Modified B-G is, however, a useful, quick screening instrument.

11.2.3. Developmental Test of Visual–Motor Integration

The Developmental Test of Visual–Motor Integration[13–15] (VMI) was developed in 1964 and was renormed in 1981 and again in 1989. The VMI was normed on 3000 children aged 2-9 to 19-8 years. The original test was applicable for children aged 4-13 years and consisted of 24 figures (two of which are derived from the B-G). Each page of the VMI is divided into six blocks: each of the top three blocks contains a design that must be copied in the box below. The reproductions are scored "pass/fail," and raw scores may be converted to developmental age equivalents, percentiles, and standard scores. Interrater reliability figures are $r = 0.90$ or above. The VMI may be individually or group administered.

The most recent revision[15] contains the 24-drawing version, which is developmentally sequenced in terms of increasing complexity. This version requires 10 to 15 min to administer and is applicable for ages 2 to 15 years. A short, 15-drawing form useful for ages 3 to 8 years is also available. The 1989 revision has revised scoring that is better at older age levels than previous versions.

The child is requested to draw figures in circumscribed areas of the page, and this feature allows for a substantial amount of structure. In addition, "pass/fail" delineations may obscure more subtle deficits. As a result, VMI performance is typically better than that of the B-G, often by as much as 2 SDs (or 18 months)[16]; correlations between the VMI and B-G are moderate, with a 45% overlap.[17] Therefore, the VMI is not interchangeable with the B-G.

The VMI manual is particularly useful in that it contains "developmental comments" in which age norms for an individual figure drawn from different authors and sources are outlined. Moreover, differentiation is made between the ages for successful imitation and copying on the first three figures (a rule of thumb is that a child can imitate a circle, vertical, or horizontal line approximately 6 months before he/she can copy it). The last section of the manual contains an excellent overview of assessment and remediation of visual–motor difficulties. The latter involves examples such as dot-to-dot exercises and those designed to remediate problems in perceptual–motor closure, recognition of similarities, and recognition of differences.

11.2.4. Minnesota Percepto-Diagnostic Test

The Minnesota Percepto-Diagnostic Test[18] (MPD) measures both visual perception and visual–motor skills. More specifically, it may assist in the differential diagnosis of learning disabilities (visual, auditory, or mixed) and in separating various behavioral problems, such as normal, emotionally disturbed, schizophrenic, or organic.[18] Two designs were derived from the B-G (circle and rotated square, and four groupings of dots that resemble an arrow), and each is presented in three different orientations, making a total of six cards. These particular designs were selected because they are most likely to be reproduced incorrectly; incorrect reproductions should also occur more frequently if the "grounds" (frames) were varied. The MPD is applicable for children aged 5 to 14 years who have normal intellect and for three age groups, (5–9, 10–15, and 16+ years) who have intelligence quotients in the 50 to 86 range. More than 4000 subjects were used for standardization. Interrater reliability varies, depending on the figure being evaluated.

The child's reproductions are scored on the basis of rotations and errors of distortion or separation. The MPD also can be used with adults. Raw scores are converted into T-scores that control for both age and IQ; these scores may also be transformed to standard deviations. In addition, "testing the limits" is encouraged when separations, rotations, or distortions occur. For example, if a rotation is present, the child should be questioned as to whether both the stimulus figure and her reproduction are "going the same way." Similarly, with a separation or distortion, the child is asked if the figures look the same or different. If the child is able to answer correctly, the problem is assumed not to be one of visual perception (input) but one of execution or integration (motor or memory, respectively).[18] A multiple-choice format may also be used for rotation errors in which the stimulus card of an incorrectly drawn figure is compared to three other cards with the stimulus in different orientations (one in the correct orientation). Correct matching would once again rule out a perceptual deficit and indicate the likelihood of an execution or integrative problem. The final limit-testing procedure is to have the child trace the MPD cards that were reproduced incorrectly. Appropriate tracings would eliminate the probability of an execution problem. If the child draws a design incorrectly but can recognize the error and trace the figure correctly, visual–motor and visual–perceptual problems can be discounted, suggesting the presence of a more complex integration (or memory) deficit.

In terms of diagnosing learning disabilities, reading-disabled children whose primary deficit is of an auditory type, reportedly obtain MPD T-scores in the 45 to 80 range. Children with a visual learning deficit score in the 31 to 44 range, whereas those having a mixed deficit ("brain damage") obtain T-scores of 0 to 30. A similar scheme is used for behavioral disturbances.[18]

The MPD test has several advantages: (1) it takes age and intelligence into consideration when evaluating the child's performance, (2) it has a recommended procedure for testing limits, and (3) it provides more insight into the *process* that goes into the child's final productions. Unfortunately, the test is underutilized at this time.

11.3. TESTS INVOLVING A MEMORY COMPONENT

11.3.1. Revised Visual Retention Test

The Benton Revised Visual Retention Test[19,20] contains three alternative forms, each consisting of ten designs. There also are four administration procedures: (1) Administration A, in which each design is exposed for 10 sec and removed, followed by immediate reproduction, (2) Administration B, where each design is exposed for 5 sec, removed, and then is followed by immediate reproduction, (3) Administration C, which requires each design to be copied by the subject, with the design remaining in the child's view, and (4) Administration D, in which each design is exposed for 10 sec, removed, and is then reproduced after a 15-sec delay. In general, most clinicians use administration A or B. Administration time is approximately 5 to 10 min.

Each design is scored as "correct" or "incorrect"; the resulting range of potential scores is 0 to 10. Scoring criteria are rather lenient because the major interest is in the child's ability to retain a visual impression (and not his/her drawing ability). Interscorer agreement is high ($r = 0.95$). Errors include omissions, additions, distortions, perseverations, rotations, misplacements, and size errors.

Norms are available for children and adults. In the former, IQ is taken into account, and adequate norms are available only for Administration A and C (for ages 7–14). The most recent revision[20] has updated norms for ages 8–adult. Therefore, the best use of this test for practitioners would be to present each card for 10 sec, remove it, and have the child reproduce the figure.

11.3.2. Memory-for-Designs Test

The Memory-for-Designs Test[21] (MFD) consists of 15 5-inch square cards with designs. Each design is exposed for 5 sec, withdrawn, and the child/adolescent is required to reproduce it. Scores from 0 to 3 are given for each reproduction, with higher scores reflecting poorer performance. Different weights are given to different types of errors. For example, orientation errors are penalized more heavily than failure to complete designs. A difference score is derived, which controls for chronological age and vocabulary level: "normal" is ≤1, "borderline" 2 to 6, and "brain damage" ≥7 error points.

Of note is the fact that both the Visual Retention Test and MFD are oriented toward "brain damage" (reflecting the type of thinking that was prevalent at the time of test development) and are not applicable for younger children. In general, normative data for children are not nearly as extensive as are those for adults. Therefore, the applicability of these two tests in regard to children is limited to a significant degree.

11.4. TESTS MEASURING VISUAL–PERCEPTUAL FUNCTION

The Motor-Free Visual Perception Test[8] (MVPT) is the most frequently used test of visual perception that does not involve graphomotor responses. The test, applicable from ages 4-0 to 8-11, consists of 36 multiple-choice items. Two types of item formats are used: (1) matching a given stimulus with one of four alternatives, or (2) selecting one of four alternatives that differs from the others. The only motor component involved is pointing. A perceptual age (based on raw scores) and a perceptual quotient are derived. The MVPT is based on a normative sample of 883 subjects. A score of ≤85 (−1 SD) is the criterion for inadequate test performance. The test requires 10 min to administer.

On the MVPT, five areas of visual perception are evaluated: (1) spatial relationships (perception of figures that are disoriented in relation to each other, such as reversals), (2) visual discrimination (ability to discriminate dominant features such as shapes or letter-like forms), (3) figure–ground (distinguish an object from its background), (4) visual closure (identify incomplete figures when only fragments have been shown), and (5) visual memory (ability to recall a visual stimulus after it is removed). Items on the MVPT are evenly divided among these categories.

The test provides useful information; however, the norms appear rather liberal, and item difficulty varies greatly within each of the five aforementioned areas of visual perception. Visual closure and visual discrimination items appear to be most valuable for the clinician. The test appears most useful for children in the 5- to 7-year age range.

11.5. SUMMARY

In addition to the specific tests described in this chapter, visual–motor and visual–perceptual functions are measured in many other test instruments. For example, visual memory is assessed with the McCarthy Scales of Children's Abilities (MSCA), the Differential Ability Scales (DAS) (Chapter 2), Stanford–Binet—Fourth Edition (SB-4), Kaufman Assessment Battery for Children (K-ABC), and the Wide-Range Assessment of

Memory and Learning (WRAML) (see Chapter 7). Visual–motor function also is evaluated on the MSCA, DAS, Wechsler Preschool, and Primary Scale of Intelligence—Revised (WPPSI-R), the Wechsler Intelligence Scale for Children—Revised (WISC-R) and WISC-III, and the WRAML (see Chapter 7). Visual–perceptual abilities are tapped on the DAS, SB-4, K-ABC, and the WISC-R/III, whereas visual–sequential skills are assessed on the WRAML, K-ABC, and WISC-III.

Practitioners may also have occasion to review or use the Rey–Osterrieth Complex Figure Test[22,23] or an alternative form, the Taylor Complex Figure Test.[24] Both tests are used to measure visual memory and hemispheric functioning in neuropsychological test batteries. On these tests, children or adults are presented with a complex figure and are asked to copy the figure as accurately as possible. The figure then is removed, and subjects are asked to reproduce the figure from memory after 20 to 40 min (without prior warning). Completed drawings may be scored qualitatively for differential copying strategies or quantitatively for accuracy of reproduction. There is evidence to suggest that although the two tests yield equivalent copy scores, the Taylor figure produced higher memory scores[25] (see Figure 11.3).

Deficits in visual–motor and visual–perceptual function may affect a child's school performance in a variety of ways. Visual–motor (execution) problems may impede development of early printing skills, thereby impairing early academic progress. Later, such deficits would interfere with

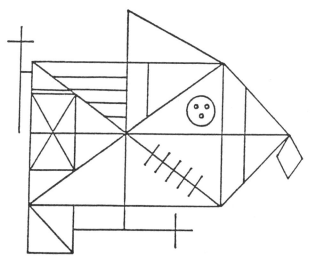

FIGURE 11.3. Rey–Osterrieth Complex Figure.

copying from the blackboard, completion of speeded paper-and-pencil tasks, or in situations where sustained graphomotor production is necessary. Subsequently, these deficits would preclude transferring thoughts to paper. Visual–perceptual deficits (input) would make letter, number, and word identification difficult and may disrupt the acquisition of reading skills. Integration problems could affect virtually any of these functions.

As alluded to earlier, attention-deficit disorders, emotional problems, and other factors may also have a negative effect on visual–motor productions. In fact, one of the first advertisements for stimulant medication included "before" and "after" medication writing samples of a child with an attention-deficit hyperactivity disorder. Impulsivity and inattentiveness have a strong influence on visual–motor function; anxiety and other emotional factors may also have a similar effect.

Finally, one must always consider the developmental processes inherent in visual–motor and visual–perceptual skills.[10] Processes evolve in the following order: (1) control of circular movement, fluidity, (2) foreground–background differentiation, organization, (3) horizontal orientation/direction, (4) verticalization, (5) diagonal orientation, and (6) differentiation and separation of figures and their parts[10] (p. 33). Unfortunately, at the present time, serial evaluations still are the only way to differentiate actual learning disabilities from maturational lags in regard to early visual–motor integrative skills.

REFERENCES

1. Bender, L., 1938, *Visual Motor Gestalt Test and Its Clinical Use. American Orthopsychiatric Association Research Monograph, 3.* American Orthopsychiatric Association, New York.
2. Koppitz, E. M., 1975, *The Bender-Gestalt Test for Young Children*, Volume 2, Grune & Stratton, New York.
3. Lesiak, J., 1984, The Bender Visual Motor Gestalt Test: Implications for the diagnosis and prediction of reading achievement, *J. School Psychol.* **22**:391–405.
4. Williams, H. J., 1983, *Perceptual and Motor Development*, Prentice-Hall, Englewood Cliffs, NJ.
5. Sattler, J. M., 1988, *Assessment of Children*, ed. 3, Jerome M. Sattler, San Diego, CA.
6. Selfe, L., 1983, *Normal and Anomolous Representational Drawing Ability in Children*, Academic Press, New York.
7. Naglieri, J. A., 1988, *Draw A Person: A Quantitative Scoring System*, The Psychological Corporation, San Antonio.
8. Colarusso, R. P., and Hammill, D. D., 1972, *Motor-Free Visual Perception Test Manual*, Western Psychological Services, Los Angeles.
9. Bender, L., 1946, *Instructions for the Use of the Visual Motor Gestalt Test*, American Orthopsychiatric Association, New York.
10. Bender, L., 1970, Use of the Visual Motor Gestalt Test in the diagnosis of learning disabilities, *J. Spec. Ed.* **4**:29–39.

11. Koppitz, E. M., 1964, *The Bender-Gestalt Test for Young Children*, Grune & Stratton, New York.
12. Brannigan, G. G., and Brunner, N. A., 1989, *The Modified Version of the Bender-Gestalt Test for Preschool and Primary School Children*, Clinical Psychology Publishing, Brandon, VT.
13. Beery, K. E., 1967, *Developmental Test of Visual-Motor Integration*, Follett, Chicago.
14. Beery, K. E., 1982, *Revised Administration, Scoring and Teaching Manual for the Developmental Test of Visual–Motor Integration*, Follett, Chicago.
15. Beery, K. E., 1989, *Developmental Test of Visual Motor Integration. Third Revision*, The Psychological Corporation, San Antonio.
16. Wright, D., and DeMers, S. T., 1982, Comparison of the relationship between two measures of visual-motor coordination and academic achievement, *Psychol. School* **19**: 473–477.
17. Cummings, J. A., and Laguerre, M., 1990, Visual–motor assessment, in: *Handbook of Psychological and Educational Assessment of Children* (C. R. Reynolds and R. W. Kamphaus, eds.), Guilford Press, New York, pp. 593–610.
18. Fuller, G. B., 1982, *The Minnesota Percepto-Diagnostic Test*, Clinical Psychology Publishing, Brandon, VT.
19. Benton, A. L., 1974, *Visual Retention Test*, The Psychological Corporation, San Antonio.
20. Benton-Sivan, A., 1991, *Benton Visual Retention Test*, ed. 5, The Psychological Corporation, San Antonio.
21. Graham, F. K., and Kendall, B. S., 1973, Memory-for-Designs Test: Revised General Manual. *Percept. Motor Skill Mon.* **Supp. 2.**
22. Rey, A., 1941, L'examen psychologique dans les cas d'encephalopathic traumatique, *Arch. Psychol.* **28**:286–340.
23. Osterrieth, P. A., 1944, Le test de capie d'une figure complexe, *Arch. Psychol.* **30**:206–356.
24. Taylor, L. B., 1969, *Psychological Appraisal of Children with Cerebral Defects*, Harvard University Press, Cambridge, MA.
25. Tombaugh, T. N., and Hubley, A. M., 1991, Four studies comparing the Rey–Osterrieth and Taylor Complex Figures, *J. Clin. Exp. Neuropsychol.* **13**:587–599.

12 ❋ Assessment of School-Performance Problems

12.1. INTRODUCTION

Typically, the primary-care physician is the first professional contacted by parents when their child experiences school difficulties. This is particularly true when disagreements exist between parents and the school system. The physician may assume several roles, depending on time and interest, each with a different level or degree of involvement. At the first level of involvement, physicians may simply refer to a psychologist for further evaluation but maintain the role of case manager. At the second level, the practitioner may elect to review existing test data, provide interpretation for parents, and plan subsequent actions. The practitioner, at the highest level of involvement, performs office screening in order to (1) develop an initial diagnostic formulation, (2) delineate the problem more precisely, (3) concisely focus referral questions, (4) alleviate parental concerns, and (5) coordinate subsequent testing and long-range planning. Variations of these three levels of intervention often occur. A thorough medical evaluation also should be performed, regardless of level of involvement. In the following discussions, it is assumed that the results of a comprehensive medical examination are not indicative of pathology.

At any level, familiarity with areas of function that must be considered in the evaluation of school-performance problems, as well as an appreciation of assessment techniques, are necessary. In the discussion that follows, etiologies for poor school performance are explored, and suggestions regarding different levels of assessment are presented.

12.2. POSSIBLE ETIOLOGIES FOR POOR SCHOOL PERFORMANCE

In general, school-performance difficulties can be grouped into four possible etiologies: (1) intellectual limitations, (2) learning disabilities, (3) attention deficits, and/or (4) behavioral disorders (Figure 12.1). The clinician's task becomes increasingly complex when these etiologies occur in combinations.

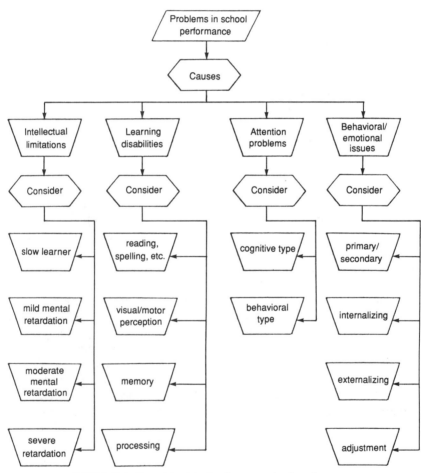

FIGURE 12.1. Potential etiologies for poor school performance.

12.2.1. Intellectual Limitations

Children with compromised intellectual abilities often experience difficulty in keeping up with the typical rate of information processing and acquisition that is encountered in the classroom. This is a particular problem in children with undiagnosed, borderline intelligence quotients ("slow learners") or high-functioning, mildly mentally retarded students (IQ scores in the 60–70 range). Often, these children are able to learn adequately if the information is presented at a slower pace and with adequate repetition. Unfortunately, most classrooms are not capable of providing this alteration in "traditional" educational programming. As a result, slow learners frequently repeat grades, and poor self-esteem and secondary emotional sequelae occur.

The primary method of determining whether or not intellectual limitation is the cause of poor school performance is to administer an intelligence test. This testing should *not* be a screen, nor should it be group administered. It is known that IQ tests may be negatively affected by learning problems (e.g., auditory processing), attention deficits, and/or emotional factors, thereby providing a false impression of compromised intellectual functioning. Moreover, children with high intellectual abilities who have similar problems may score in the average range, but, in reality, this is not in keeping with their true potential. Administration of intelligence tests also is valuable in the delineation of specific areas of strengths and weaknesses, such as abstract reasoning, processing speed, verbal/performance discrepancies, or attention problems. The data may also provide various clues that are indicative of areas that require further exploration. In addition to providing an IQ score, intelligence testing provides a method of evaluating different aspects of school functioning.

12.2.2. Learning Disabilities

It is apparent that learning disabilities (LDs) can have a profound adverse effect on school performance. In addition to the more specific learning disabilities in academic subjects such as reading recognition, reading comprehension, spelling, or mathematics, other, more subtle problems may exist. These include deficits in memory (visual, auditory, or both), visual–motor integration or visual perception (see Chapter 11), processing speed, abstract concept formation, sequential processing, or auditory processing. These types of learning problems are much more difficult to identify, frequently occur in combination, and do not fit into many school systems' learning-disability eligibility requirements. However, these problems often are the underlying basis for more apparent reading, spelling, or mathematics difficulties.

12.2.3. Attention Deficits

Attention problems frequently are underdiagnosed.[1] Not uncommonly, they mimic auditory processing dysfunction (or vice versa) or memory problems. Attention problems may affect visual–motor skills, the child's ability to comprehend lengthy verbal input, or performance of multistep operations. Attention deficits may cause the child to make multiple, careless errors and can disrupt: (1) initial input of information, (2) processing of information once it is received, or (3) execution of a response. Children with attention deficits may demonstrate hypoarousal, whereby they can focus their attention for periods of time if the task is challenging and stimulating. However, with routine, sustained, or less interesting tasks (which, unfortunately, often are found in the classroom), attention may wane. The end result is a history of inconsistent performance coupled with perplexed parents and teachers. A variation in this profile is the child who may be able to "fire up" and perform adequately for weeks or even months at a time (typically because of consequences or threats of consequences for poor academic performance). However, the intense effort required to focus, organize, and perform academically takes its toll. The end result is a "burnout" phenomenon, whereby the child simply stops trying, and grades plummet. Often, there is adequate performance during the initial quarter of the school year, followed by a gradual decline (often attributed to "the holidays"), resulting in marked deterioration by the last quarter.

12.2.4. Behavior Problems

Behavioral/emotional problems such as acting out, anxiety, depression, or impulsivity may adversely affect school performance. A primary challenge for the clinician is to determine whether the behavioral/emotional problems represent a primary pathology or are secondary to school difficulties. Frequently, disruptive classroom behavior, refusal to do schoolwork, and/or inattentiveness are maladaptive reactions to the learning difficulties or the frustration caused by lack of academic success. These behaviors, in effect, may be "face-saving," allowing the child to take some measure of control over an actual or perceived uncontrollable situation. A comprehensive, focused history is imperative, inasmuch as learning disabilities do not occur suddenly (although they may become more apparent as work demands increase). Emotional issues should also be explored if there are reports that the child completes homework but often "forgets" to turn it in. In the later grades, "learned helplessness" or similar phenomena may cause a student to suppress all efforts, prompting the complaint that the child "could do the work if he/she tried." Also included in delineation of the differential diagnosis are depressive, anxiety, conduct, oppositional/defiant, or psychotic disorders. All these disorders can negatively influence academic performance.

12.3. AREAS OF ASSESSMENT

As suggested in the previous chapters, information from five areas of assessment should be considered in the evaluation of poor school performance: (1) intelligence (IQ), (2) academic achievement, (3) attention, (4) behavior, and (5) visual–motor/visual–perceptual function. In the discussion that follows, algorithms (decision trees) are presented. Depending on the findings in each area of assessment, different considerations and recommended courses of action are presented.

12.3.1. Evaluation of Intelligence

An algorithm for the evaluation of IQ is presented in Figure 12.2. The first step in the evaluation of IQ test data involves determination of discrepancies or deviant test-score patterns (1) between verbal and performance scores (e.g., Wechsler Intelligence Scale for Children[2]—WISC-R/WISC-III), (2) between sequential versus simultaneous processing (e.g., Kaufman Assessment Battery for Children[3]—K-ABC), (3) test factors (e.g., WISC-III), or (4) specific areas of function (e.g., Stanford–Binet-IV[4]—SB-4). If scores are comparable, with little variation between subtests and no unusual behaviors noted during testing, but IQ scores are low, then intellectual limitation should be considered as the underlying cause of the poor school performance. If these criteria are met but the IQ score is in the average range or better, then other etiologies should be explored (left side of decision tree).

If discrepancies between IQ scores, significant differences between test factors, or large subtest variations are noted, further consideration of learning disabilities is necessary. The IQ score should be reviewed with caution, because large discrepancies may invalidate the overall IQ esti-

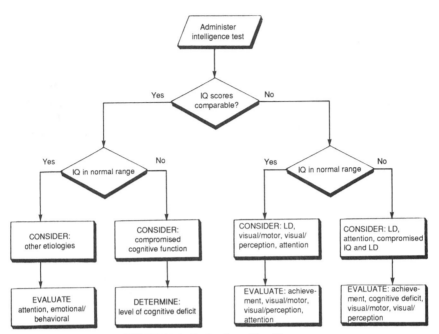

FIGURE 12.2. Evaluation of intelligence.

mate. If verbal/performance[2] or sequential/simultaneous[3] differences are noted, consideration of factor indices (e.g., verbal comprehension, perceptual organization)[2] is necessary, as is the assessment of visual–motor/visual–perceptual functioning and visual and auditory memory. If no discrepancy is found in overall verbal/performance scores, the possibility of more circumscribed learning disabilities (auditory processing, processing speed) and attention problems should be evaluated (right side of decision tree). Essentially, the same etiologies should be considered, regardless of whether or not the IQ score falls in the average range, because this may simply reflect the degree of the interfering problem (e.g., LD, attention, etc.).

In order to obtain an estimate of IQ, the Kaufman Brief Intelligence Test[5] (K-BIT; see Chapter 7) or the Peabody Picture Vocabulary Test—Revised[6] (PPVT-R; see Chapter 3) may be administered in the office. Because of limitations of these screening instruments, the clinician can be more confident if average or above-average performance is obtained (thereby ruling out intellectual deficiencies). Below-average performance may be affected by various factors (particularly in the case of the PPVT-R); therefore, a low score does not necessarily mean that the child has intellectual limitations. Reciprocally, many group tests administered by the school may overestimate IQ. It is critical that previous psychological testing data be reviewed, and these should be current (i.e., obtained within the last 3 years).

If testing has not been performed, IQ testing should be administered by a psychologist. Specific IQ tests are recommended for different age groups and situations (see Chapters 6 and 7) and for evaluation of specific deficits.

12.3.2. Evaluation of Academic Achievement

Estimates of the child's current levels of academic performance are necessary. Although standardized group testing data obtained at various grades are useful, they can be affected negatively by a variety of factors (disinterest, comprehension problems, inattention). High scores, however, generally tend to discount the plausibility of an academic learning disability. An algorithm for academic achievement is found in Figure 12.3.

As was discussed in Chapter 6, the primary criterion for determination of learning disabilities is the presence of a "discrepancy" (1) between current grade placement and level of academic performance, (2) between aptitude (IQ) and achievement, or (3) between achievement levels in different areas of academics (intra-achievement).

The first step in the evaluation process is a comparison of the child's level of academic achievement with his/her current grade placement. However, there are several caveats to be considered in this procedure. Grade equivalents are the weakest descriptive measure obtained for this type of testing. Standard scores, percentiles, and stanines are better measures (see Chapter 8). Second, the degree of discrepancy necessary to qualify for special education services varies, depending on the school district (usually one or two grades). It should be noted that a one-grade delay in the primary grades is more significant than a similar delay at later grades (Chapter 8).

The next step is to evaluate whether academic achievement is significantly below (i.e., discrepant from) the child's IQ score. If there is no difference between the two, and all academic areas are comparable, the possibility of compromised IQ being the underlying cause for poor performance is raised. This should be verified by further consideration of IQ testing. On the other hand, when the student's academic performance is below grade level, and academic achievement is below his/her aptitude, then learning disabilities should be considered, regardless of whether or not all achievement areas are comparable (left side of decision tree). The

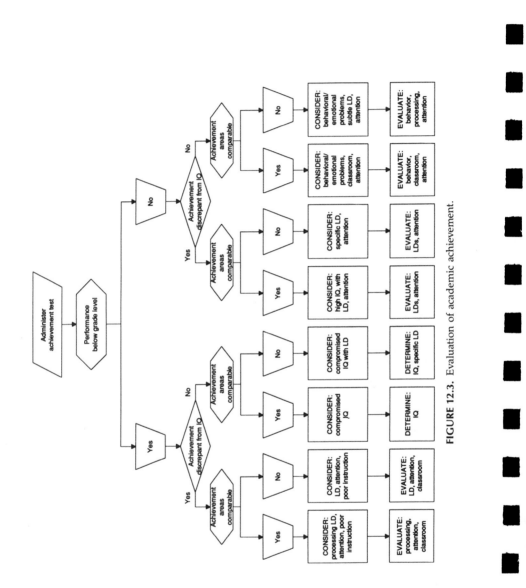

FIGURE 12.3. Evaluation of academic achievement.

practitioner also should consider attention deficits and/or poor classroom instruction.

In the event that the child's academic performance is not below grade level but is below what would be predicted from the IQ score, then the possibility of an intellectually advanced student with either learning disabilities or an attention problem should be considered. The situation in which academic achievement is not below grade level or discrepant from IQ but the child is performing poorly academically warrants consideration of behavioral/emotional issues (with or without LDs) or poor classroom instruction (right side of decision tree).

The primary-care physician is encouraged to perform screening of academic achievement in the office, from which both quantitative and qualitative information should be obtained. The Wide-Range Achievement Test-Revised[7] (WRAT-R) or the WRAT-3, the Kaufman Test of Educational Achievement Brief Form[8] (KTEA), or Wechsler Individual Achievement Test Screener[9] are highly useful as quick screens. The Boder Test of Reading/Spelling Patterns[10] can also be used if concerns focus specifically on reading or spelling problems. Selected subtests from the Peabody Individual Achievement Test-Revised[11] (PIAT-R), Woodcock–Johnson Psychoeducational Battery-Revised[12] (WJ-R), or the Wechsler Individual Achievement Test[9] (WIAT) (e.g., listening comprehension) may be utilized as well. However, it is recommended that these test instruments be administered in their entirety if at all possible.

12.3.3. Assessment of Attention/Concentration

In Chapter 9, checklists or rating scales, computerized assessment, and psychometric testing were recommended as techniques to be used in the evaluation of attention or concentration problems. A schematic decision tree for this type of evaluation is found in Figure 12.4.

Adjunctive information is important in the evaluation of attention problems. Therefore, rating scales are recommended as the first step in the evaluation of this particular problem area (see Chapter 10). Narrow-band or unidimensional scales would be appropriate if completed by both parents and teachers and accompanied by the School Situations Questionnaire.[13,14] In all probability, teacher rating scales would be more sensitive to primary attention problems, whereas parent checklists would be more apt to detect activity and behavior problems.[15] If an attention disorder is suspected, computerized assessment should be administered regardless of whether or not the checklists were positive. Positive findings on rating scales, computerized assessment, and psychometric testing (left side of

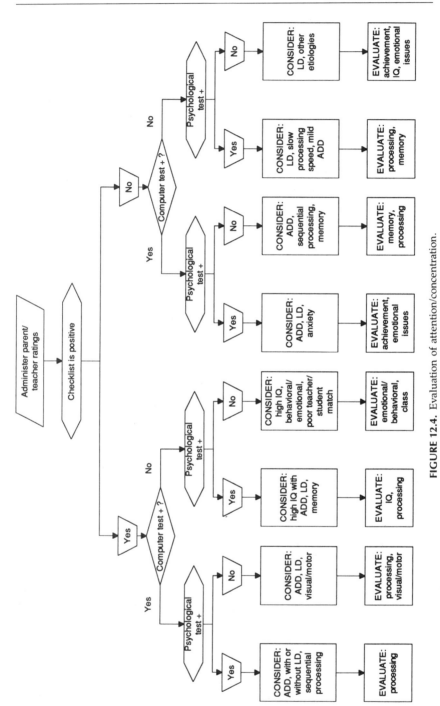

FIGURE 12.4. Evaluation of attention/concentration.

decision tree) suggest attention-deficit disorders, with or without learning disabilities. If checklists and psychometric testing data are positive but computerized assessment is not, the possibility of a child with above-average intelligence and ADD, other learning disabilities, or memory problems should be considered. When only checklists are positive, the differential diagnosis should include consideration of a behavioral/emotional problem or a poor teacher–student match.

In situations in which computerized assessment is positive but rating scales are not, consider ADD without hyperactivity, a learning problem, or both (regardless of whether or not psychometric testing is positive). If psychometric testing data are positive, anxiety should also be considered. Additional testing with the Wide-Range Assessment of Memory and Learning[16] (WRAML; see Chapter 7) would be very helpful.

When rating scales, computerized assessment, and psychometric testing data are not suggestive of ADD, other etiologies should be explored, particularly internalizing emotional issues such as anxiety or depression. If only psychometric testing is positive, a learning disability is possible (right side of decision tree).

Practitioners should obtain teacher, parent, and situation (home, school) rating scales. Computerized assessment (CPT; see Chapter 9) is helpful but is usually not available in most practices. The use of telephone or fax transferral of CPT data to generate a report from a third party is convenient. However, this procedure is not recommended because this practice may overlook qualitative information and behaviors that are important. Short-term visual and auditory memory tasks are helpful and can be drawn from a variety of sources such as Levine's neurodevelopmental tests,[17] the WRAML,[16] or similar instruments.

In addition to qualitative indicators obtained during testing (impulsivity, activity, out-of-seat behavior, inattentiveness), the WISC-III Freedom from Distractibility Index and the Processing Speed Index[2] as well as WRAML short-term memory and learning subtests (see Chapter 7) should be reviewed. Children with attention-deficit disorders often hide these indicators over a short or moderate period of time. Therefore, more intensive testing, typically lasting for several, 1-hr sessions, often enables the clinician to observe the child's more "typical" behavior.

12.3.4. Assessment of Behavior

Rating scales enable measurement of emotional functioning, personality, characteristic behaviors such as attention or activity, and adaptive functioning (see Chapter 10). Unidimensional or "narrow-band" rating scales as well as multidimensional or "broad-band" scales are available. The former are more restricted in the types of behavior that can be evaluated (e.g., attention, hyperactivity). Conversely, the latter allow for wider sampling of behaviors such as withdrawal, anxiety, depression, delinquency, or aggression. Although lengthy, comprehensive questionnaires provide more information; however, there is a general reluctance by some parents and teachers to complete this type of form. A schematic decision tree for the evaluation of behavior problems is found in Figure 12.5.

It is suggested that narrow-band (unidimensional) rating scales be used first in the assessment of problems in school performance. If the rating scale is positive only for attention or hyperactivity problems, a broad-band instrument may not be necessary, depending on the results of other areas of testing. However, when scores on narrow-band unidimensional checklists are extreme or are suggestive of behavioral problems, more detailed evaluation with multidimensional scales is recommended. Positive findings on both types of scales are strongly suggestive of ADHD (possibly with oppositional features) or significant behavioral/emotional

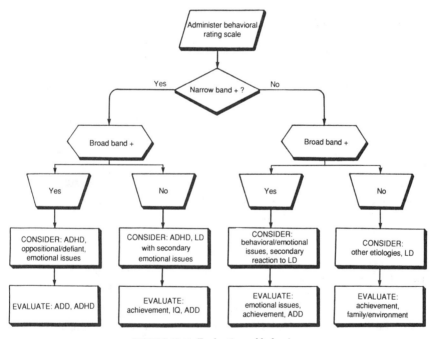

FIGURE 12.5. Evaluation of behavior.

issues (left side of decision tree). Further evaluation of emotional function is necessary. Positive findings only on attention and hyperactivity indices (these can also be obtained on subscales of broad-band instruments) with no indicators of other behavioral problems are more indicative of ADHD, although secondary emotional issues may also be present.

If *neither* narrow-band nor broad-band scales are positive for attention, hyperactivity, or other behavioral problems, then the clinician should consider other etiologies for the school problem (right side of decision tree). In the case of positive findings only on emotional indicators of broad-band scales, the clinician is advised to consider behavioral/emotional difficulties, perhaps secondary to learning disabilities.

Unidimensional scales such as the ADD-H Comprehensive Teacher Rating Scale[18] (ACTeRS) or the Connors Teacher and Parent Scales[19] may be used first. If extreme scores or problems in all areas are found, then use of a multidimensional scale such as the Child Behavior Checklist[20] (CBCL), the Personality Inventory for Children[21] (PIC), or the Behavior Assessment System for Children[22] (BASC) is recommended. A clinical interview is suggested, including the child and the parents. Often in the evaluation of behavioral problems, information is obtained solely from the parents; however, the child can provide much information as well. If emotional or behavioral difficulties are indicated, evaluation by a psychologist or child psychiatrist of the child's emotional functioning is recommended. This evaluation generally will include drawings and other projective techniques.

12.3.5. Assessment of Visual–Motor and Visual–Perceptual Function

Visual–motor and visual–perceptual function may have a significant, adverse effect on a child's school performance (see Chapter 11). It is recommended that a test of visual–motor function be administered in the diagnostic work-up. A schematic decision tree to evaluate this area is found in Figure 12.6.

A visual–motor integrative test should be administered first in the assessment procedure. Clinicians should be cognizant of the distinction between deficits in perception, execution, or integration (Chapter 11), and testing of limits should be considered. Regardless of whether the child's visual–motor production is below chronological age, a measure of visual perception also should be employed. When both visual–motor *and* visual–perceptual abilities are deficient, visual–motor, visual–perceptual, and/or visual–motor integrative dysfunctions should be considered; concomitant ADD also should be evaluated. Visual–motor problems can exist in the

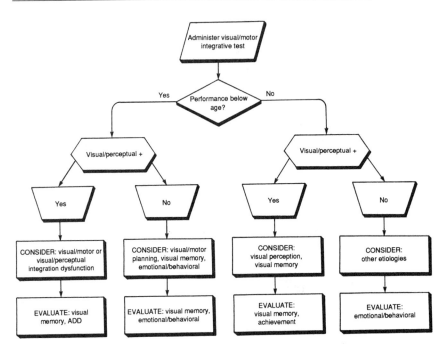

FIGURE 12.6. Evaluation of visual–motor/visual–perceptual function.

presence or absence of visual–perceptual dysfunctions, visual–motor planning deficits, emotional/behavioral dysfunction (see Koppitz's[23] scoring criteria), or problems in visual memory (left side of decision tree).

Even if visual–motor problems are not apparent, it is helpful to assess visual perception. Visual–perceptual deficits may be found in the absence of visual–motor problems. If this occurs, considerations should include visual–perceptual deficits or visual–memory problems. Additional information should also be reviewed, including the simultaneous subtests of the Kaufman Assessment Battery for Children[3] (K-ABC), the WISC-III[2] block design, coding, and object assembly, and performance-related subtests of the WPPSI-R[24] and the Stanford–Binet-4.[4] If neither visual–motor nor visual–perceptual deficits are found, this area probably is not a major factor in the child's school performance problems, and other areas should be considered.

Screening for visual–motor and visual–perceptual function in the office is relatively easy; the Bender-Gestalt,[25] Minnesota Percepto-Diagnostic Test,[26] or Developmental Test of Visual–Motor Integration[27] are brief and can be administered by the physician or nurse with a minimal amount of training. With younger school children, copying letters and numbers and possibly a dictated sentence also is helpful. The Wide-Range Achievement Test–Revised[7] spelling subtest (see Chapter 8) or the written expression subtest of the Peabody Individual Achievement Test–Revised (see Chapter 8) is similarly useful.

The second level of assessment generally includes evaluation of visual memory with tests such as the Memory for Designs Test,[28] the Benton Visual Retention Test[29] (see Chapter 11), or Wide-Range Assessment of Memory and Learning.[16] The accrued data then can be reviewed in conjunction with subtest scaled scores obtained from administration of intelligence tests.

12.4. PROBLEM CASES

To reiterate, the evaluation of a child with school difficulties should include assessment of intelligence, academic achievement, attention/concentration, behavior, and visual–motor/visual–perceptual functioning. In the following hypothetical cases, a $7\frac{1}{2}$-year-old male, currently enrolled in the second grade, is referred for evaluation because of poor academic achievement. Vision, hearing, and gross neurological function are within normal limits; medical evaluation reveals no pathologies. The evaluation instruments described in the preceding chapters were utilized to determine whether a deficit or problem (indicated by a "+") was found.

Case 1. Positive findings are noted in IQ, academic achievement, and visual–motor/visual–perceptual function. Depending on the nature of the positive findings, the possibility of cognitive deficiency or a learning disability should be entertained. Figures 12.2, 12.3, and 12.6 should be reviewed for clarification of the types of dysfunction found (Table 12.1).

TABLE 12.1. Hypothetical Cases Involving Problems in School Functioning

Case	Intelligence	Academic achievement	Attention/ concentration	Behavioral	Visual–Motor/ Visual–Perceptual
1	+[a]	+	−	−	+/−
2	−	+	+	+	+
3	+	−	−	−	+
4	+	+	+	+	+
5	+	+/−	+/−	−	−
6	−	−	+	+	−

[a]A + denotes a positive finding.

Case 2. Positive findings in the areas of academic achievement, attention/concentration, behavior, and visual–motor/visual–perceptual function are found. Consideration of an attention-deficit disorder (with behavioral manifestations), learning disability, and/or emotional problems is suggested. Figures 12.3 to 12.6 should be reviewed. The likelihood of an emotional etiology increases if the history reveals an abrupt decline in academics and/or the presence of major life stresses (Table 12.1).

Case 3. Intelligence testing and visual–motor/visual–perceptual dysfunction are indicative of problems. Perceptual or visual–motor dysfunction should be considered, particularly if there is a significant verbal/performance IQ discrepancy, favoring the former (see Figures 12.2 and 12.6).

Case 4. Difficulties are found in all areas. In such situations, cognitive deficiency, learning disabilities, ADD, behavioral problems, or some combination should be considered. In this type of profile, review of specific test scores within each of the five areas of evaluation (all figures) is necessary for clarification.

Case 5. Deficits in IQ-testing data are noted, although the results of academic achievement and attention/concentration evaluation are questionable. A specific learning disability, perhaps of an auditory sequencing type, may be present. Subtests measuring this area of processing as well as the *type* of reading, spelling, and mathematics errors should be reviewed (see Figures 12.2 to 12.4). Attention problems also require further assessment (Table 12.1).

Case 6. Positive findings in the attention/concentration and behavioral areas are obtained. Attention-deficit disorder (probably with hyperactivity) and/or behavioral problems are likely. The latter possibility is more probable, given negative findings in IQ and academic achievement (see Figures 12.4 and 12.5).

12.5. SUMMARY

In primary-care medicine, it is not uncommon to be called upon to evaluate children and adolescents with school problems. If the presenting problems primarily involve poor grades, and these are not accompanied by obvious behavioral problems, referral to an educational diagnostic team is likely.[30] Conversely, if the child acts out behaviorally, referral to a mental health professional is typical. Practitioners often must determine if emotional and behavioral difficulties are causing academic problems, or whether the emotional/behavioral issues are the result of the academic problem.[30] Therefore, in addition to evaluation of the child, the practitioner must consider family and environmental issues.[31] Family issues may involve (1) parenting problems, (2) marital problems, (3) employment, and (4) siblings. Environmental issues may include (1) peer problems, (2) values systems, and (3) school.[31]

The clinical assessment of problems in school performance is complicated, and there often are multiple explanations for these difficulties. In fact, it is rare that any specific problem is caused by a single factor.[31] Concerted efforts by the physician, parents, teachers, and other professionals are essential in an effective diagnostic approach.

REFERENCES

1. Kelly, D. P., and Aylward, G. P., 1992, Attention deficits in school aged children and adolescents: Current issues and practice, *Pediatr. Clin. North Am.* **39**:487–513.
2. Wechsler, D., 1991, *Manual for the Wechsler Intelligence Scale for Children-III*, The Psychological Corporation, San Antonio.
3. Kaufman, A. S., and Kaufman, N. L., 1983, *Interpretive Manual for the Kaufman Assessment Battery for Children*, American Guidance Service, Circle Pines, MN.
4. Thorndike, R. L., Hagen, E. P., and Sattler, J. M., 1986, *Guide for Administering and Scoring the Fourth Edition*, Riverside Publishing Co., Chicago.
5. Kaufman, A. S., and Kaufman, N. L., 1990, *Kaufman Brief Intelligence Test*, American Guidance Service, Circle Pines, MN.
6. Dunn, L. M., and Dunn, L. M., 1981, *Peabody Picture Vocabulary Test—Revised*, American Guidance Service, Circle Pines, MN.
7. Jastek, S., and Wilkenson, G. S., 1984, *Wide-Range Achievement Test—Revised*, Jastek Associates, Wilmington, DE.
8. Kaufman, A. S., and Kaufman, N. L., 1985, *Kaufman Test of Educational Achievement*, American Guidance Service, Circle Pines, MN.
9. The Psychological Corporation, 1992, *Manual for the Wechsler Individual Achievement Test*, The Psychological Corporation, San Antonio.
10. Boder, E., and Jarrico, S., 1982, *The Boder Test of Reading-Spelling Patterns*, Grune & Stratton, New York.
11. Markwardt, F. C., 1989, *Peabody Individual Achievement Test—Revised*, American Guidance Service, Circle Pines, MN.
12. Woodcock, R. W., and Johnson, M. B., 1989, *Woodcock–Johnson Psycho-Educational Battery—Revised*, DLM Teaching Resources, Allen, TX.
13. DuPaul, G. J., 1991, *The Home and School Situations Questionnaire—Revised: Normative Data, Reliability, and Validity*, unpublished manuscript, University of Massachusetts Medical Center, Worcester.
14. Barkley, R. A., and Edelbrock, C., 1987, Assessing situational variation in children's problem behaviors: The home and school situations questionnaires, in: *Advances in Behavioral Assessment of Children and Families*, Volume 3 (R. J. Prinz, ed.), JAI Press, Greenwich, CT, pp. 157–176.
15. Biederman, J., Keenan, K., and Farone, S. V., 1990, Parent-based diagnosis of attention deficit disorder predicts a diagnosis based on teacher report, *J. Am. Acad. Child Adoles. Psychiat.* **29**:698–701.
16. Sheslow, D., and Adams, W., 1990, *Wide-Range Assessment of Memory and Learning. Administration Manual*, Jastek Associates, Wilmington, DE.

17. Levine, M. D., 1985, *Examiner's Manual. Peeramid*, Educators Publishing Service, Cambridge, MA.
18. Ullmann, R. K., Sleator, E. K., and Sprague, R. L., 1988, *Manual for the ADD-H Comprehensive Teacher's Rating Scale*, Metrotech, Champaign, IL.
19. Conners, C. K., 1989, *Manual for Conners Rating Scales*, Multi-Health Systems, North Tonawanda, NY.
20. Achenbach, T. M., 1991, *Manual for the Child Behavior Checklist/14–18 and 1991 Profile*, Department of Psychiatry, University of Vermont, Burlington.
21. Wirt, R. D., Lachar, D., Klinedinst, J. E., Seat, P. D., and Broen, W. E., 1984, *Personality Inventory for Children*, Western Psychological Services, Los Angeles.
22. Reynolds, C. R., and Kamphaus, R. W., 1992, *BASC. Behavior Assessment System for Children Manual*, American Guidance Service, Circle Pines, MN.
23. Koppitz, E. M., 1975, *The Bender-Gestalt Test for Young Children, Volume 2*, Grune & Stratton, New York.
24. Wechsler, D., 1989, *WPPSI-R Manual*, The Psychological Corporation, San Antonio.
25. Bender, L., 1946, *Instructions for the Use of the Visual Motor Gestalt Test*, American Orthopsychiatric Association, New York.
26. Fuller, G. B., 1982, *The Minnesota Percepto-Diagnostic Test*, Clinical Psychology Publishing, Brandon, VT.
27. Beery, K. E., 1989, *Developmental Test of Visual–Motor Integration, Third Revision*, The Psychological Corporation, San Antonio.
28. Graham, F. K., and Kendall, B. S., 1973, Memory-for-Designs Test: Revised General Manual, *Percept. Motor Skill. Monogr.* **Suppl. 2**.
29. Benton-Sivian, A., 1991, *Benton Visual Retention Test, Fifth Edition*, The Psychological Corporation, San Antonio.
30. Silver, L. B., 1993, Introduction and overview to the clinical concepts of learning disabilities, *Child. Adoles. Clin. North Am.* **2**:181–192.
31. Ostrander, R., 1993, Clinical observations suggesting a learning disability, *Child. Adoles. Clin. North Am.* **2**:249–263.

13 ❋ Additional Considerations

13.1. INTRODUCTION

The challenges involved in the provision of comprehensive primary care to children and their families have changed considerably. In addition to the "traditional" medical concerns, developmental, cognitive, and emotional issues must be addressed. As was stated at the outset, the purpose of this book is to address these changes by providing the practitioner with germane information and useful techniques.

Rather than simply providing the primary-care physician with a voluminous listing of developmental and psychological tests, this book is couched within the framework of two of the most common behavioral/developmental problems: (1) suspected developmental delay and (2) difficulties in school performance. Within this context, various tests and suggestions for screening, assessment, and formulation of the differential diagnosis are provided. In addition, the review focuses on strengths and weaknesses inherent in each of the screening and evaluation tests. Each section culminates in applications and illustrative cases.

The primary-care physician also must address differentiating "normal" and "abnormal" emotional development. The physician again usually is the professional of first contact when parents have concerns about individual differences and temperament,[1] childhood depression,[2] mother–infant interactions,[3] or anxiety disorders.[4] Questions regarding discipline,[5] family function,[6] or types of parenting[3] also typically are raised by parents. A useful outline for informal evaluation of emotional functioning in infants and young children was provided by Greenspan.[7] This schema includes general parenting patterns as well as age-specific child tendencies. History taking, clinical interviews, observation of parent–child interaction, and developmental testing[7] are suggested as means of obtaining relevant data. Unfortunately, emotional/behavioral issues typically are not adequately addressed in many pediatric and family practices.

13.2. CAVEATS AND ISSUES IN DEVELOPMENTAL ASSESSMENT

When evaluating young children, clinicians often are faced with the dilemma of differentiating static versus evolving dysfunction. The term "evolving" is used instead of "progressive" because the latter suggests a worsening diagnostic picture. A "static" dysfunction, such as cerebral palsy or severe mental retardation, typically is the result of central nervous system trauma. The presentation of static dysfunction may be variable, as in the case of hypotonia, which often evolves into a phase of normal tone and then progresses to hypertonia. This example underscores the need for serial evaluation. In contrast, mild mental retardation presents more of an "evolving" picture in that it becomes increasingly apparent as the child ages, and it can become more pronounced if the child resides in an understimulating environment. Change in degree of dysfunction also depends on the area of function that is assessed. For example, there is evidence that mild motor problems tend to improve over time, whereas cognitive functioning is not as "self-righting,"[8] particularly in the face of a nonstimulating environment.[9,10] Therefore, one area of dysfunction may not necessarily be predicted by the assessment of the child's performance in other areas of developmental function.

Several interesting pitfalls in developmental diagnosis have been raised by Blasco.[11] As was indicated in the initial chapters, practitioners may be lulled into a false sense of security by a child who manifests normal gross motor development. Discrepancies between levels of motor and cognitive development often occur, particularly in mild mental retardation. In fact, in one patient series, one-half of the severely mentally retarded children were able to ambulate by 18 months (a mild delay), and one-third walked by 15 months of age (the upper limit of normal).[12] Clinicians also must attend to both gross and fine motor development. Once again, fine motor functions may be divergent from gross motor skills, with the former being more sensitive to subtle delays.

Blascoe outlined the pitfall of establishing impressions based on superficial physical appearances. Readers are undoubtedly sensitive to the issue that dysmorphic features do not always equate with developmental delays; however, the reverse is not necessarily true.[13] More specifically, a pretty or handsome child who displays a pleasant temperament, average motor skills, but who also manifests developmental delays may not be identified simply because he/she does not "look" delayed.

Practitioners are not generally familiarized in their training with delays in prelinguistic milestones, congenital deafness, or lesser degrees of hearing impairment. Hearing deficits can be evaluated below 1 year of age,[14] and health care providers should be aware that the risk criteria for congenital hearing impairment include: (1) a positive family history, (2) congenital infection, (3) head and neck malformations, (4) very low birth weight, (5) hyperbilirubinemia, (6) bacterial meningitis, or (7) severe asphyxia.[15] To compound matters further, language and problem-solving skills are the best predictors of later cognitive functioning; however, these same functions can be negatively affected by poor oral–motor and fine motor skills.

Correction for prematurity is another major issue.[16,17] A general "rule of thumb" is that correction, i.e., subtracting the weeks of prematurity from the child's chronological age, should be applied up to 2 years of age. Although there is a fair degree of agreement that correction is necessary over the first year of life, later correction is controversial. Obviously, 12 or more weeks correction would generally inflate scores; however, not correcting at all would place the child at a distinct developmental disadvantage. It is not clear what should be done for the child born at 36 weeks gestational age: no correction, correction for 1 week, or correction to 40 weeks. It is most likely that some type of correction formula will evolve, based on the child's gestational age at birth and chronological age. Perhaps correction should be up to 36 and not 40 weeks. However, until this issue is resolved (if ever), it is often useful for the clinician to obtain both corrected and uncorrected scores. Obviously, if the corrected score is above average and the unadjusted score is average, the physician can be fairly confident that development looks appropriate at this time. If, however, even with a large correction, the child barely falls in the average range (scores ≤90), and the uncorrected score is indicative of delays, then caution must be exercised (with careful surveillance). This situation is made more complex if the child has a fragile medical condition or has been hospitalized frequently.

As was indicated in Chapter 5, physicians often are reluctant to convey "bad news" to parents, instead minimizing the situation and hoping that the child "will grow out of it." Although the physician may initially bear the brunt of the parents' anger at the presentation of such news, the long-term consequences of withholding this information are much worse.[18] These include the parents' resentment for not "telling the truth," increased parental guilt for not "doing something" earlier, and delay in the initiation of interventions. Many physicians eschew "labeling" a child; unfortunately, such labeling often is a necessary requirement in obtaining services. This issue should be clarified for parents. Interventions do appear to be beneficial; however, efficacy depends on the child's diagnosis, age of initiation of intervention, type of program, duration, family involvement, and how efficacy is measured.[19,20]

Therefore, in dealing with suspected developmental delays, health care providers should bear in mind three clinical principles[21]: (1) developmental screening instruments should identify children with developmental disabilities that would not be recognized without their use; (2) intervention programs for children having preschool developmental problems are beneficial[19,20]; and (3) a growing system is becoming available to deal with developmentally delayed preschool children.[22] Several ramifications emanate from these principles: (1) children with more mild cognitive or language deficits are most likely to be the ones identified with developmental screening instruments; (2) there is a considerable amount of data that support the positive educational and therapeutic benefits of early intervention (particularly in children with mild cognitive and/or language problems), and (3) PL 99-457 and the more recent PL 102-119 have mandated that states develop systems to identify and manage children with developmental problems.[21]

13.3. CAVEATS AND ISSUES IN EVALUATION OF SCHOOL PROBLEMS

Learning disabilities, without question, have a significant impact on the quality of a child's later life. Unfortunately, learning disabilities are not as easily defined as is mental retardation, with diagnosis of LDs usually being made when the child is older (see Chapter 6). As a result, the child with learning disabilities typically has experienced more opportunities in which he/she has been unsuccessful, thereby increasing the risk of adverse psychological sequelae.

Pediatricians traditionally focus on hyperactivity or attention-deficit disorders as their primary concept of LD.[23] As a result, this influx of learning disabilities, or the "new morbidity,"[24] is perplexing to physicians, in part because it is not caused by specific organic disease,[25] nor is it easily remedied after the diagnosis is made. The issue is compounded because a variety of new laws have been passed over the past two decades to deal with problems in school-aged children (see Purvis for a more detailed history and review).[25]

Consequently, practitioners must be well versed in mental retardation, hearing impairment, serious emotional disturbance, physical impairment, and learning disabilities. Moreover, primary-care physicians need to have knowledge of the steps necessary to access special services and advocacy. In general, before evaluation for special services can be initiated, it must be documented that the child's needs are not being met adequately in the regular classroom. At this more informal level, a multidisciplinary team might make a classroom observation, interview teachers, have an academic screening performed by a learning-disabilities teacher, and review the child's academic history and progress.[26] The data obtained from this first step will determine whether a more comprehensive evaluation is required. Unfortunately, "academic screening" may overlook subtle learning disabilities or assume that average achievement is appropriate in a gifted but learning-disabled student.

The formal evaluation typically is initiated by school personnel (e.g., teacher or principal), but it can also be requested by a parent via communication with the teacher, principal, or director of special education. Parents must give written approval for more detailed evaluation or a "second opinion." Formal stages of the process include a comprehensive evaluation, development of an Individual Educational Plan (IEP; which is based on the test data and developed in a meeting between school personnel and the parents), determination of delivery method of instruction (pull-out or self-contained), and periodic reevaluation of progress and services. There are specified time frames between when the request for evaluation is received and when it must be completed. School systems must acknowledge testing data obtained by other professionals and indicate how they will handle these data. The schools do not, however, have to accept these data and instead can perform additional testing of their own. Knowledge of services and programs available within the practitioner's state and community is essential. However, state and local educational systems have their individual idiosyncracies in evaluation and management.

Physicians also must be current in regard to medication and educational interventions,[27] as well as "fad" treatments such as diets, colored glasses, eye–hand coordination exercises, and neuromotor programming.[28] Defining a child's strengths is at least as important as elucidating weaknesses, particularly in light of subsequent interventions and self-concept issues.

13.4. "PEARLS"

The final section of this chapter focuses on various techniques that are useful in explaining learning disabilities and medication and answering questions regarding later outcomes and interventions. These concluding comments are directed primarily to problems in school performance. Many of these "pearls" resulted from sharing information with colleagues in the course of various conferences and workshops. These anonymous

contributors are acknowledged for their wisdom and clinical acumen—
with best wishes for their continued success in working with young
patients and their families.

13.4.1. Explaining Learning Disabilities

Often, a diagnostic evaluation is itself a therapeutic intervention for
the child. For example, by explaining what a learning disability is (under-
scoring the student's strengths, and suggesting that the primary reason for
the evaluation is to make school "better" for the child), the practitioner
frequently places the child at ease and helps to enhance self-esteem.
Similarly, clarifying for the parents that the child's problems in school
performance are not the result of being "lazy" or "immature" (a favorite
term in educational circles that will be discussed later) is highly beneficial.
Third-person techniques such as "sometimes kids who have problems
reading think they're dumb," are very useful.

13.4.1.1. Circuit Board

In this high-tech age, children are familiar with the concept of circuit
boards or computer chips. Noting that the brain is analogous to a computer circuit board (or chip) is useful; certain circuits run talking, whereas
others control walking, math, reading, etc. Sometimes certain circuits or
parts of the chip don't work quite right (depending on the child's disability), whereas other parts function quite well. The "programmer" (namely,
the child) has to figure out ways to get around the circuit that doesn't
work.

13.4.1.2. Racing Car

In this analogy, the child is compared to an expensive racing car, such
as a Ferrari or Lamborghini. The car looks good, contains good parts, is
fast and impressive, but at present, the car is not going as fast as it could
because the fuel injector isn't functioning properly. The "mechanics" have
to figure out how to fix the fuel injector as best they can, because it is a
special part that cannot simply be taken out and replaced. The brakes,
steering, electrical system, and other parts of the car function perfectly.
Once the car is repaired, it will run very fast once again, but it might need
to use a few extra horsepower (i.e., extra effort) to do so. This is a
"language" that is readily appreciated by children.

13.4.2. Learning Disability Explanations for Parents

Parents often ask for an explanation of the causes for LDs. Frequently, they recall a perinatal difficulty or some other historical marker as the potential etiology. It is important to explain that the brain is rarely, if ever, "perfect," and that virtually everyone has some imperfections. Unfortunately, imperfections in a child's brain may be more apparent because of the demands imposed by academic challenges. The parent may be advised that it is virtually impossible to identify the "spot" in the brain that causes the problem.

Another question posed by most parents relates to an LD problem persisting as the child grows older. More specifically, they question whether the child will overcome the disability. Obviously, no one can predict the future, and outcome is dependent on the *type* and *severity* of dysfunction.[29] However, indicating a belief that the child can be a productive member of society is most important. As children grow older, their interests migrate toward areas in which they are "good"; therefore, outside of school, LDs would be less apparent or impairing. It is important to emphasize that an individual simply does not "get over" a learning disability but, instead, learns compensatory strategies to circumvent the problem.

Parents similarly are confused by what they can do to address the problem. The practitioner should caution parents that their zeal to remediate the learning disability by intensive home instruction can be counterproductive. After a difficult day at school in which areas of deficit are addressed repetitively, children do not want to be subjected to the same exercises once again at home. Although extra work at home may be beneficial (depending on what is provided by the school system), the bulk of the remediation effort should be accomplished at school or with tutors. Families should be encouraged to be supportive, accepting, and to have their interactions directed toward extracurricular activities such as sports, hobbies, and recreational pursuits. This approach allows for more "quality time" and prevents the focus of family interactions from centering on the stressful area of academics. Parents are encouraged/urged to channel their energies into advocacy efforts for their child.

13.4.3. Grade Retention

Physicians should anticipate that parents will seek advice about grade retention. There are few clear rules for making this decision and even less research on the long-term outcome after grade retention.[30] In fact, there is increasing evidence that grade retention or even delaying school entry are not the best interventions for children with learning problems.[31] Retention often is presented in the context of the child being "immature." However, this term is defined with the scientific rigor of a ouija board. Generally, retention is not a useful intervention. Unfortunately, as was discussed in previous chapters, many children whose intelligence scores fall in the slow learner range repeat grades. In some cases, if the child is found to be severely behind classmates academically, is not mentally deficient, and does not have a learning disability or attention problem, then grade retention may be necessary. However, this should be regarded as an exception. Children with attention-deficit disorders are at increased risk for grade retention, with as many as 25% to 35% of these children being retained at least once before entering high school.[32]

Alterations in the child's educational program are essential, even if grade retention occurs. If this intervention is *absolutely* necessary, it should happen in kindergarten or first grade. Repeating a later grade can be emotionally devastating for the child and is a distinct threat to developing self-esteem. Careful assessment of the child's present levels of academic achievement is critical in any deliberations relating to grade retention.

An analogy can be made that repeating a grade is like running a race with a broken leg. The child comes in last place and is informed that by running the race again, he/she will do better. However, nothing has been done to repair the broken leg. Many school systems have "transitional" or "developmental" early elementary grades in which the information is presented at a much slower pace. After completion of this grade, the child may then be able to enter the same grade in a regular classroom. This approach helps in some cases, but this type of program usually is limited to kindergarten and first grade (the assumption being that the child will somehow improve so as to not need this type of intervention in later grades).

A critical issue in early grade retention involves accurate differentiation of academic problems attributable to delays in *maturational readiness* (a so-called nativist viewpoint) from those caused by underlying *dysfunction* (i.e., ADD or LD). Many teachers endorse the "nativist" approach and therefore recommend that the child repeat a grade so as to have "another year to grow up."[30,33] When early grade retention is being considered by parents, practitioners need to consider (1) academic status, (2) physical size and chronological age, (3) the child's emotional maturity, (4) remedial services that can be offered, and (5) the style and expectations of the next grade teacher.[30] In kindergarten, if the child's overall developmental levels are significantly below chronological age and grade, his/her birthday is close to the cut-off, and physical size is small, retention *may* be appropriate.[30] However, if retention ultimately is recommended (and even when it is merely being considered), one must critically evaluate the type of teaching approach that was employed previously (and, unsuccessfully at that), and what changes can be made this time to enhance teaching effectiveness.[30]

13.4.4. Explaining Attention-Deficit Disorders to Children

The child's brain can be compared to the command center of a spaceship or submarine. The command center can place the rest of the ship on alert or can tell the crew to be on the lookout for certain things such as other ships, planets, or asteroids. Moreover, the command center can keep the crew alert by periodically rebroadcasting orders or messages. Unfortunately, for the child with ADD, any one of these functions may be working improperly. The task of intervention is to help the command center be better able to control the ship once again. Several other techniques are found in the literature, such as Levine's command cockpit.[34] Using the term *attention problem* versus the usual nomenclature is also advised.

13.4.5. Explaining Attention-Deficit Disorders to Parents

Parents have a myriad of misconceptions about attention-deficit disorders, many of which are promulgated by the lay press or television. Indicating that there is both a behavioral and a cognitive form[27] is helpful, as is discussing many of the associated features and apparent inconsistencies.

Practitioners may suggest that although the exact causes of ADD have not been clearly defined, there is evidence for a possible biochemical etiology. In particular, the executive parts of the brain that control the focusing of attention and that inhibit activity and tuning in to extraneous stimuli are not working efficiently. Treatment involves "firing up" these executive parts (e.g., frontal lobes)—often by increasing the amount of particular neurotransmitters or "brain chemicals" (dopamine and norepinephrine). This explanation format is also appropriate for use with older school-aged children or adolescents with ADD. Parents and children similarly may appreciate the analogy of "needing a cup of coffee in the morning in order to get going"; stimulant medication serves a similar purpose. The practitioner should anticipate many questions regarding side effects, the continued need for medication, and related issues. Review of the article by Kelly and Aylward[27] is helpful in this regard. In general, ADD persists in 50% to 60% of individuals, although the motor component subsides by adolescence. However, the negative aspects of ADD routinely are more apparent in school than in the workplace; moreover, the creativity and energy that often are inherent in ADD may later work to the individual's benefit.

13.4.6. Explaining the Use of Medication to Children

Children have many questions about medication as well. The practitioner should emphasize that the major positive changes the child may encounter following the use of medication result from the child's efforts rather than simply the medication per se. Medication helps the child to help himself/herself. Effort is needed, however, because the medication is not magical. Medication may allow children to think before doing and helps them to focus. The expectation should be transmitted to the child that at some point he/she will learn how to do these things without the use of medication. However, at this time, medication will be necessary in order to learn what to do.

The use of medication can also be compared to glasses. Glasses can help a person who has poor vision to see; however, this can be accomplished only if the individual wants to see better. If he keeps his eyes closed, glasses simply will not be useful.

Physicians should carefully monitor parents' statements concerning medication. Sometimes the covert message is given that the child cannot function without it or that he/she has to behave, lest the medication will be doled out. Obviously, neither of these messages is appropriate.

In summary, the importance of developmental and school-related problems cannot be minimized, nor should they be considered any less significant than organic or physical disorders. Both of these problems may have long-term influences that affect the quality of life. How the physician handles these problems often determines the extent of these influences.

REFERENCES

1. Carey, W. B., 1992, Temperament issues in the school-aged child, *Pediatr. Clin. North Am.* **39**:569–584.
2. Aylward, G. P., 1989, Child/adolescent depression. Guidelines for office management,

in: *Developmental-Behavioral Disorders*, Volume 2 (M. I. Gottlieb and J. E. Williams, eds.), Plenum Press, New York, pp. 1–13.

3. Aylward, G. P., 1992, Behavioral and developmental disorders of the infant and young child: Assessment and management, in: *Behavioral Pediatrics* (D. E. Greydanus and M. L. Wolraich, eds.), pp. 81–97, Springer-Verlag, New York.

4. Bernstein, G. A., 1990, Anxiety disorders, in: *Psychiatric Disorders in Children and Adolescents* (B. D. Garfinkel, G. A. Carlson, and E. B. Weller, eds.), W. B. Saunders, Philadelphia, pp. 64–83.

5. Howard, B. J., 1991, Discipline in early childhood, *Pediatr. Clin. North Am.* **38**:1351–1370.

6. Hutter, M. J., 1991, Office evaluation and management of family dysfunction, *Adoles. Med. State Art Rev.* **2**:303–312.

7. Greenspan, S. I.,1991, Clinical assessment of emotional milestones in infancy and early childhood, *Pediatr. Clin. North Am.* **38**:1371–1386.

8. Aylward, G. P., Gustafson, N., Verhulst, S. J., et al., 1987, Consistency in diagnosis of cognitive, motor, and neurologic function over the first three years, *J. Pediatr. Psychol.* **12**:77–98.

9. Aylward, G. P., 1990, Environmental influences on the developmental outcome of children at risk, *Inf. Young Child* **2**:1–9.

10. Aylward, G. P., 1992, The relationship between environmental risk and developmental outcome, *J. Dev. Behav. Pediatr.* **13**:222–229.

11. Blasco, P. A., 1991, Pitfalls in developmental diagnosis, *Pediatr. Clin. North Am.* **38**:1425–1438.

12. Hreidarsson, S. J., Shapiro, B. K., and Capute, A. J., 1983, Age of walking in the cognitively impaired, *Clin. Pediatr.* **22**:248.

13. Lock, T. M., Shapiro, B. K., Ross, A., et al., 1986, Age of presentation in developmental disability, *J. Dev. Behav. Pediatr.* **7**:340.

14. Bess, F. H., and McConnell, F. E., 1981, Measurement of auditory function, in: *Audiology, Education, and the Hearing Impaired Child*, C. V. Mosby, St. Louis.

15. Roizen, N., 1991, Neurosensory hearing loss, in: *Developmental Disabilities in Infancy and Childhood* (A. J. Capute and P. J. Accardo, eds.), P. H. Brookes, Baltimore.

16. Aylward, G. P., 1988, Issues in prediction and developmental follow-up, *J. Dev. Behav. Pediatr.* **9**:307.

17. Blasco, P. A., 1989, Preterm birth: To correct or not to correct, *Dev. Med. Child. Neurol.* **31**:816.

18. Kaminer, R. K., and Cohen, H. J., 1988, How do you say, "Your child is retarded?" *Contemp. Pediatr.* **5**:36.

19. Shonkoff, J. P., and Hauser-Cram, P., 1987, Early intervention for disabled infants and their families: A quantitative analysis, *Pediatrics* **80**:650.

20. Bennett, F. C., and Guralnick, M. J., 1991, Effectiveness of developmental intervention in the first five years of life, *Pediatr. Clin. North Am.* **38**:1513–1528.

21. Casey, P. H., and Swanson, M., 1993, A pediatric perspective of developmental screening in 1993, *Clin. Pediatr.* 209–212.

22. Blackman, J. A., Healy, A., and Ruppert, E. S., 1992, Participation by pediatricians in early intervention: Impetus from Public Law 99-457, *Pediatrics* **89**:98–102.

23. Hagerman, R. J., 1984, Pediatric assessment of the learning-disabled child, *J. Dev. Behav. Pediatr.* **5**:274–284.

24. Casey, P. H., Bradley, R. H., Caldwell, B. M., et al., 1986, Developmental intervention: A pediatric clinical review, *Pediatr. Clin. North Am.* **33**:899–953.

25. Purvis, P., 1991, The public laws for education of the disabled—the pediatrician's role, *J. Dev. Behav. Pediatr.* **12**:327–339.

26. Whelan, R. J., 1988, *Special Education Procedural Due Process*, The University of Kansas, Lawrence.
27. Kelly, D. P., and Aylward, G. P., 1992, Attention deficits in school-aged children and adolescents: Current issues and practice, *Pediatr. Clin. North Am.* **39:**487–513.
28. Levine, M. I., 1987, An update on learning disabilities, *Pediatr. Ann.* **16:**105–108.
29. Shaywitz, S. E., Escobar, M. D., Shaywitz, B. A., et al., 1992, Evidence that dyslexia may represent the lower tail of a normal distribution of reading disability, *N. Engl. J. Med.* **326:**145–150.
30. Shelton, T. L., 1993, To retain or not to retain: That is the question, *ADHD Rep.* **1:**6–8.
31. Cameron, M. B., and Wilson, B. J., 1990, The effects of chronological age, gender, and delay of entry on academic achievement and retention: Implications for academic redshirting, *Psychol. School* **27:**260–263.
32. Szatmari, P., Offord, D. R., and Boyle, M. H., 1989, Correlates, associate impairments, and patterns of service utilization of children with attention deficit disorders: Findings from the Ontario child health study, *J. Child Psychol. Psychiat.* **30:**205–218.
33. Smith, M. L., and Shepard, L. A., 1988, Kindergarten readiness and retention: A qualitative study of teachers' beliefs and practices, *Am. Ed. Res. J.* **25:**307–333.
34. Levine, M., 1990, *Keeping a Head in School*, Educators Publishing Service, Cambridge, MA.

❀ **Appendixes**

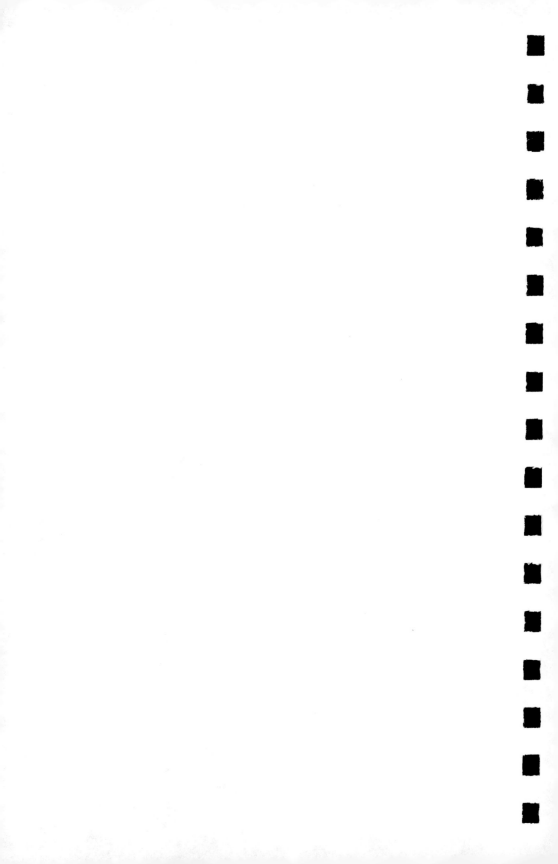

A ❃ Sources for Selected Screening and Evaluation Instruments

Publisher	Test	Acronym	Area(s) assessed[a]
The Psychological Corporation 555 Academic Ct. San Antonio, TX 78204	Basic Achievement Skills Individual Screener	BASIS	ACH
	Bayley Infant Neurodevelopmental Screen	BINS	D
	Bayley Scales of Infant Development/Bayley II	BSID	D
	Boder Test of Reading–Spelling Patterns	Boder	Ach
	Boehm Test of Basic Concepts	—	L
	Cattell Infant Intelligence Scale	—	D
	Comprehensive Test of Adaptive Behavior	—	Adap
	Developmental Test of Visual–Motor Integration	VMI	V/M
	Devereux Behavior Rating Scale	—	B
	Differential Ability Scales	DAS	D, I
	FirstSTEP Screening Test for Evaluating Preschoolers	FirstSTEP	D
	Gesell Developmental Schedules	—	D
	McCarthy Scales of Children's Abilities	MSCA	D, I
	Miller Assessment for Preschoolers	MAP	D
	Preschool Language Scale-3	PLS	L
	Revised Visual Retention Test	—	V/M
	Wechsler Individual Achievement Test	WIAT	Ach

Publisher	Test	Acronym	Area(s) assessed[a]
	Wechsler Intelligence Scale for Children—Revised/Wechsler Intelligence Scale for Children-III	WISC-R WISCIII	I
	Wechsler Preschool and Primary Scale of Intelligence-Revised	WPPSI-R	I
American Guidance Service Circle Pines, MN 55014-1796	Behavior Assessment System for Children	BASC	B
	Children's Attention and Adjustment Survey	CAAS	A/C
	Kaufman Assessment Battery for Children	KABC	I
	Kaufman Brief Intelligence Test	KBIT	I
	Kaufman Test of Educational Achievement	KTEA	Ach
	Peabody Individual Achievement Test—Revised	PIAT-R	Ach
	Peabody Picture Vocabulary Test—Revised	PPVT-R	L
	Preschool Attainment Record	PAR	B
	Vineland Adaptive Behavior Scales	VABS	Adap
DLM Teaching Resources One DLM Park Allen, TX 75002	Battelle Developmental Inventory	BDI	D
	Inventory for Client and Agency Planning	ICAP	Adap
	Scales of Independent Behavior	SIB	Adap
	Woodcock–Johnson Psychoeducational Battery—Revised	WJR	Ach
Riverside Publishing Co. 8420 Bryn Mawr Avenue Chicago, IL 60631-3476	Gates MacGinitie Reading Tests	—	Ach
	Stanford–Binet—Fourth Edition	SB-4	I
Western Psychological Services 12031 Wilshire Blvd. Los Angeles, CA 90025	Arizona Articulation Proficiency Scale-R	AAPS-R	L
	Developmental Profile II	—	D
	Louisville Behavior Checklist	LBC	B
	Motor-Free Visual Perception Test	MVPT	V/M
	Personality Inventory for Children	PIC	B
Hawthorne Educational Services P.O. Box 7570 Columbia, MO 62505	Attention Deficit Disorders Evaluation Scale	ADDES	A/C

Publisher	Test	Acronym	Area(s) assessed[a]
PRO-ED 8700 Shoal Creek Blvd. Austin, TX 78758	AAMD Adaptive Behavior Scales Early Language Milestone Scale	— ELMS/ELMS-2	Adap L
Clinical Psychology Publishing Co. 4 Conant Square Brandon, VT 05733	Minnesota Percepto-Diagnostic Test Modified Version of the Bender-Gestalt Test for Preschool and Primary School Children	MPD —	V/M V/M
Behavioral Science Systems Minneapolis, MN	Minnesota Child Development Inventory Minnesota Child Development Preschool Inventory	MCDI MCDI-PS	Adap, B Adap, B
Jastek Associates P.O. Box 3410 Wilmington, DE 19804-0250	Wide-Range Achievement Test—Revised Wide-Range Assessment of Memory and Learning	WRAT-R WRAML	Ach A/C, M
Kent Developmental Metrics Kent, OH 44240-3178	Kent Infant Development Scales	KIDS	D
Denver Developmental Materials, Inc. P.O. Box 6919 Denver, CO 80206-0919	Denver Developmental Screening Test/Denver II Prescreening Developmental Questionnaire	DDST/DDST-II PDQ	D D
Multi-Health Systems, Inc. 908 Niagara Falls Blvd. N. Tonawanda, NY 14120-2060	Conners Continuous Performance Test Conners Parent and Teacher Rating Scales	CCPT CPRS/CTRS	A/C A/C, B
Metritech, Inc. 111 N. Market St. Champaign, IL 61820	ADD-H Comprehensive Teacher Rating Scale	ACTeRS	A/C, B
Educators Publishing Service 75 Moulton St. Cambridge, MA 02138	Aggregate Neurobehavioral Health and Education Review	ANSER	B, A/C
GSI Publications P.O. Box 746 DeWitt, NY 13214	Gordon Diagnostic System	GDS	A/C

[a]Abbreviations: D, developmental; I, intelligence; Ach, achievement; B, behavioral; L, language; A/C, attention/concentration; V/M, visual–motor/visual–perceptual; Adap, adaptive; M, memory.

B ❃ Additional Sources for Rating Scales

Author	Instrument	Acronym	Area assessed
Thomas M. Achenbach, Ph.D. Department of Psychiatry University of Vermont Burlington, VT 05401	Child Behavior Checklist	CBCL	Behavior/attention
Russell A. Barkley, Ph.D. Department of Psychiatry University of Massachusetts Medical Center 55 Lake Avenue North Worcester, MA 01655	Home Situations Questionnaire School Situations Questionnaire	HSQ/SSQ	Attention
C. Keith Conners, Ph.D Department of Psychiatry Duke University Medical Center Durham, NC 27710	Conners, Loney, and Milich Questionnaire	CLAM	Attention
George J. DuPaul, Ph.D. Department of Psychiatry University of Massachusetts Medical Center 55 Lake Avenue North Worcester, MA 01655	Home Situations Questionnaire- Revised School Situations Questionnaire- Revised	HSQ-R SSQ-R	Attention
Craig S. Edelbrock, Ph.D. Department of Psychiatry University of Massachusetts Medical Center 55 Lake Avenue North Worcester, MA 01655	Child Attention/ Activity Profile	CAP	Attention

Author	Instrument	Acronym	Area assessed
Sheila M. Eyberg, Ph.D. Department of Clinical Psychology University of Florida Box J-165, JHMHC Gainesville, FL 32610	Eyberg Child Behavior Inventory	ECBI	Behavior
Philip C. Kendall, Ph.D. Department of Psychology Temple University Weiss Hall, Fourth Floor Philadelphia, PA 19122	Self-Control Rating Scale	SCRS	Attention
Jan Loney, Ph.D. Department of Psychiatry Putnam Hall-South Campus SUNY at Stony Brook Stony Brook, NY 11794-8790	IOWA Conners	IOWA	Attention
William Pelham, Ph.D. Department of Psychiatry Western Psychiatric Institute and Clinic 3811 O'Hara Street Pittsburgh, PA 15231	Swanson, Nolan, and Pelham Rating Scale-R	SNAP-R	Attention
Herbert C. Quay, Ph.D. Program in Applied Social Sciences University of Miami P.O. Box 248074 Coral Gables, FL 33124	Revised Behavior Problems Checklist	R-BPC	Behavior/attention

✽ Index